（汉英对照）
Chinese–English Edition

实用中医病案学基础

Basis on Practical Medical Records of Traditional Chinese Medicine

主　编——陈晓云　刘　萍

副主编——王　骁　傅勤慧

主　审——陈湘君　苏　励　Charles Savona–Ventura

Editor–in–chief——Chen Xiaoyun　Liu Ping

Deputy Editor–in–chief——Wang Xiao　Fu Qinhui

Lead Trial——Chen Xiangjun　Su Li　Charles Savona–Ventura

上海科学技术出版社

Shanghai Scientific & Technical Publishers

图书在版编目（ＣＩＰ）数据

实用中医病案学基础 = Basis on Practical
Medical Records of Traditional Chinese Medicine :
汉英对照 / 陈晓云, 刘萍主编. -- 上海 : 上海科学技
术出版社, 2022.1
　　ISBN 978-7-5478-5204-0

Ⅰ. ①实… Ⅱ. ①陈… ②刘… Ⅲ. ①中医治疗法－
病案－汉、英 Ⅳ. ①R242

中国版本图书馆CIP数据核字(2021)第259577号

实用中医病案学基础
Basis on Practical Medical Records of Traditional Chinese Medicine
主编　陈晓云　刘　萍

上海世纪出版(集团)有限公司
上 海 科 学 技 术 出 版 社　出版、发行
(上海市闵行区号景路 159 弄 A 座 9F－10F)
邮政编码 201101　www.sstp.cn
上海盛通时代印刷有限公司印刷
开本 787×1092　1/16　印张 15.5
字数 280 千字
2022 年 1 月第 1 版　2022 年 1 月第 1 次印刷
ISBN 978－7－5478－5204－0／R·2236
定价：168.00 元

本书如有缺页、错装或坏损等严重质量问题,请向工厂联系调换

本书围绕中医各种常用病案的特点和书写规范,介绍了中医病案学的发展背景、现代应用和写作要求,包括中医病案学的历史与发展、中医学写作与"诚信"、中医辨证分析在病案中的应用;列举了常用病案的写作形式和规范,包括门诊病历、住院病历、临床案例报告、平行病历、中国中医诊断国家标准、国际疾病分类及编码系统,同时介绍了中医药会议报告书写、研究设计写作等。

本书内容丰富、图文并茂、深入浅出、实例典型,既可作为高等中医院校中医留学生教材,又可供各类从事中医药国际教育的教师参考。

This book is an academic monograph on the characteristics and writing standards of various commonly used medical records of traditional Chinese medicine. It introduces developing background and modern practice, writing requirements of medical record of traditional Chinese medicine, including the history and development of traditional Chinese medicine medical record science, the construction of "integrity" in Chinese medicine writing, and the application of syndrome differentiation analysis in medical records. It also lists the writing forms and norms of common medical records, including outpatient medical records, inpatient medical records and case reports from clinical records, parallel case records, the Chinese national standard of TCM diagnosis, international disease classification and coding system etc. Moreover, meeting report and poster, research design writing were introduced inside.

This book is rich in content, graphic and illustrated by reading plain text together with viewing picture. It is easy to master through simple terms and typical examples. It can not only be used as teaching materials for overseas students in colleges or universities of traditional Chinese medicine, but also be used as a reference for teachers engaged in international education of traditional Chinese medicine.

内容提要

Content summary

前言 —— Preface

近年来，随着中医药对外交流的不断发展与扩大，来华学习中医的留学生规模逐年增加，加强和完善留学生教育已经成为现代中医教育中的一个重要组成部分。古人云，文以载道。中医药学术的研究与发展离不开相应病案的记录和阐明。有道无文，行而不远；有文无道，华而不实。规范中医病案书写对于中医药学术的发展与传播起着至关重要的作用。

随着时代的发展，中医病案书写不再局限于传统医案形式，文体形式不断变化和丰富。对于留学生而言，汉语基础比较薄弱，文化背景不同，要想写出规范的中医病案有一定的难度。写作没有捷径，但有自己的规范和要求。然而，单一理论知识学习比较枯燥，且实用性不高。通过理论知识讲解、实例阐述、各类病案写作练习、情境练习等多种方式相结合，可以充分激发学生学习热情，调动学生写作潜能，在不断地思考与训练中，熟悉和掌握各种中医病案书写规范，提高中医病案写作能力。

目前适合留学生学习中医病案书写的相关教材比较少，这就使我们萌发了撰写一部中医病案学专著的想法，详细介绍中医病案学的历史沿革、各种中医病案书写规范以及中医临床诊疗术语和双重编码系统。于是，经过整理编撰便有了这本书的诞生。希望本书的出版，对中医留学生，以及各中医专业的医学生学习规范书写中医病案有所帮助。

本书付梓之时，相关全英文课程已在上海中医药大学国际教育学院全英文班连续讲授了4年，获得了学生们的认可和喜爱。在全体任课老师、助教、指导专家和学员的共同努力下，课程日趋完善。但作为一本新的教学用书难免有所疏漏，真诚地希望国内外同道给予我们意见、建议和指导，帮助我们在不久的将来进一步完善这本著作。本书编撰过程得到了上海市名中医苏励教授和上海中医药大学附属龙华医院中医内科学教研室相关专家的大力支持，英文部分有幸得到了上海中医药大学国际教育学院韩丑萍老师的悉心指导以及马耳他大学中医中心主任查尔斯·撒蒙纳·万图拉教授的斧正，在此特别致谢！

编者
2021年9月

In recent years, with the development and expansion of foreign exchanges of TCM, the number of oversea students who studying TCM in China would have been increasing year by year. Strengthening and improving the training of oversea students has become one of the most important parts in modern TCM education. As the ancients said, the words are used to express the Way(道, Dao, the general rules of universe). The academic research and development of TCM is inseparable from the recording and clarification of corresponding medical records. The Way without words is hard to spread, the words without Way is flashy and useless. Standardized writing of TCM record plays a vital role in the development and dissemination for TCM.

With the development of times, the forms of TCM records were not only limited to the traditional types, they are constantly changing and enriched. For foreign students, due to relatively lower Chinese language level and different cultural background, it is difficult for them to write standardized records of TCM. There is no shortcut for TCM records, but the practice itself has its own rules and requirements. However, just to study theoretical knowledge is boring and not very practical. Through the combination of theoretical knowledge explanation, case discussion, various medical record writing exercises and situational practice, etc., the learning enthusiasm of students can be fully stimulated, their writing potential can be mobilized. With continuous thinking and training, they are going to get familiar with various TCM records and master them. And their ability of writing TCM records shall be significantly improved.

At present, there are very few related textbooks which are suitable for oversea students to learn the writing of TCM records, that makes the idea of writing a monograph on TCM records come to our mind. A book to introduce the history of TCM records, rules and regulations on TCM record writing, terminology of TCM practice and the double coding system for diagnosis. And then, after a pile of arrangement and edit, the book came to birth. Hopefully, it could facilitate the study process of overseas TCM students and the other medical students who are willing to improve writing skills on TCM records.

Before the publishing of the book, the related English courses have been continuously offered to students in the English class from the college of International Education, Shanghai University of TCM for 4 years, and have been approved and loved by our students. With the co-efforts of our lecturers, teaching assistants, consultants and students, the course is becoming better and better. However, as a new textbook and reference, it is inevitable that there could be some omissions. Sincerely, we hope that experts at home and abroad could give us opinions, suggestions and guidance to help us further improve this book in the near future. The compilation process of this book was strongly supported by Professor Su Li, the Shanghai famed TCM doctor and experts from the teaching and research department of Internal Chinese Medicine, Longhua Hospital. Fortunately, the English version of this book has been revised by both Professor Han Chouping from College of International Education, Shanghai University of TCM and Professor Charles Savona Ventura, the head of TCM center, University of Malta. Last but not least, we would like to express our sincere gratitude to all the doctors, professors and people who have contributed to this book. Your efforts are critical to make this happen.

Editor-in-chief

Sept. 2021

Chapter One

History and Development of TCM Records / 8

Appendix Two

Appendix Three

第一章 中医病案学的历史与发展

无论你有多聪明，记忆力有多好，做记录是记住所有重要信息的最有效方式之一。特别是如果你是一名医生，面对上千名不同的患者，准确地记住一切信息是不可能的。因此，医疗记录对每位医生来说都是非常重要的。

一、中医病案溯源

医疗记录是患者病情如何发生、发展、诊断和治疗的过程总结。

1. 早期阶段（商代至隋代） 我们今天所能找到的最早的中医记录是商代兽骨和龟甲上的甲骨文（图1-1）。在这些珍贵的古代文献中，发现了21个与健康相关条文的记录。公认的最早的中医病案记录是2170年前汉代成书的《史记·扁鹊仓公列传》中的25条病案记录（图1-2）。在晋代葛洪所著的《肘后备急方》和隋代巢元方的《诸病源候论》中也有一些医案记载。而我国最早发明和使用病历的，是汉初的内科医生淳于意。行医时，淳于意会把患者的姓名、地址、病症、药方、诊疗日期等一一记录下来，治愈的、死亡的无一例外。长此以往，淳于意发现这种记录对于诊断和治疗裨益颇多，于是将其命名为"诊籍"。

2. 繁荣阶段（唐代至明清） 唐宋以来，中医病案记录越来越受欢迎。宋代许

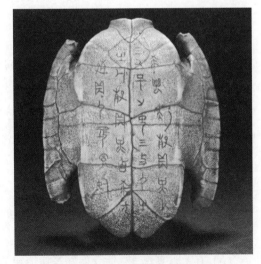

图1-1　商代兽骨和龟甲上的甲骨文
（图片来源 California Asian Art Auction Gallery）

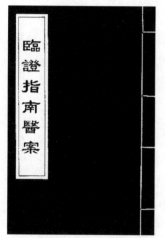
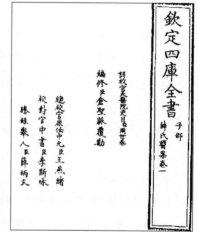

图 1-2　《史记》《临证指南医案》
（图片来源 http://ctext.org/library）

叔微所著《伤寒九十论》是历史上第一本中医病案记录专著。在明清时期，医生越来越重视总结出版医案记录。在这时期涌现了许多著名的代表作，如明代薛己的《薛氏医案》和清代叶天士的《临证指南医案》。如今的中医从业者仍然可以从这些古代专著中获取有用的经验。1584 年，明代吴崑在其代表作《脉论》中总结了分七个部分的病案记录格式：

（1）就诊时间，患者姓名和籍贯。

（2）望诊和问诊的结果。

（3）疾病发生的时间，疾病的原因，患者的情绪状态以及相关的既往史。

（4）初步诊断，治疗和结果。

（5）有无恶寒、恶热，饮食偏好等病情相关的临床表现，是否有跟时间变化相关的病情加剧。

（6）诊断及相关病因，治疗方法。

（7）详细处方，治疗原则和解释。

另外吴崐还强调了医生签名的重要性。他总结的格式为现代中医记录打下了坚实的基础。明代江瓘所著《名医类案》和清代魏之琇所著《续名医类案》是中医病案专著的杰出文献。时至今日，仍被中医从业者广泛阅读和研究。

由于朝代的限制，这些病案专著都是个人实践的产物，并未广泛地遵循格式的标准化。

二、现代医学病历起源

在 1900 年之前，现代医学病例书写并没有统一的标准格式。事实上，除了检查脉搏之外，许多医生甚至没有直接接触过他们的患者。医学和占星术是同源学科，与占星家不同，医生执医过程中并不需要持笔。他们的许多诊断都依靠患者的肤色、尿液和其他排泄物，因此可记录的内容并不丰富。医生保存书面记录的习惯晚于占星家，但在性质上更加多样化。它们大致分为三类：受中世纪晚期欧洲发展的记录形式所影响，最基本的是客户名单及其对治疗或处方的支付清单；而古希腊医案则出现了有关治疗的记载，并在 14 世纪和 15 世纪被广泛应用。其中包括对患者饮食和食谱的建议，治愈结果的记录，尸体解剖或外科医生学习的笔记，这种方法在 16 世纪得到了扩展和成倍增长；随着这一趋势的发展，医生开始记录诊疗过程中所"观察"的内容（图 1－3）。在随后的几十年中，病例记录开始在医院中流传并保存，标志着更为系统和客观的医疗实践的开端。

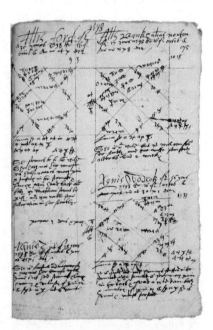

图 1－3 福尔曼和纳皮尔的案例簿
他们的记录早于现代医疗记录，具有重要的意义（《从纸莎草到电子平板的图片：临床医疗记录的简史和数字时代的课程》）

三、现代中医病案的发展

中华人民共和国成立后，成立了许多中医医院。但当时医疗记录全都是按照西医的模式进行的。1982 年，中华中医药学会（CACM）起草了《中医病案书写格式和要求》第一版。

在草案试行后,又作了修改调整。1988 年,国家中医药管理局(SATCM)要求中华中医药学会在全国范围内由专家对草案进行磋商和修改,最终确定了该国家标准。1991 年,《中医病案书写规范》正式发布实施。2002 年《医疗事故处理条例》通过实施。作为该法律的补充,发布了《中医、中西医结合病历书写基本规范(试行)》。

现行的《中医病历书写基本规范》为 2010 版。由国家卫生和计划生育委员会(NHFPC)以及国家中医药管理局(SATCM)起草的,于 2002 年 7 月 1 日生效,2010 年修订。该规范主要包含了 4 个方面内容:中医病历书写通则,门急诊病历书写内容与要求,住院病历书写内容及要求,打印病历要求。住院病历书写内容各国要求不同,大致包括入院记录(24 小时内完成),首次病程记录(8 小时内完成),首次查房记录(48 小时内完成),主治医师日常查房记录,阶段小结等。中医对于现病史的记录,除了记录疾病的发生、发展、入院前诊疗经过这些现有症状外,还应基于"十问歌",饮食、睡眠、二便,记录中医病因病机和治疗。中医院诊断目前实行双诊断,即西医诊断和中医诊断。诊疗计划也包含中西医两个方面。

附:中医用药度量衡发展历史

方剂中,药物的用量一般以最新版《中华人民共和国药典》为指导,根据药物性质、剂型、配伍关系和患者的年龄、体质、病情以及季节的变化而酌定。目前的中药剂量是借鉴古代经典著作、结合长期的临床实践逐步演变换算而来。由于年代久远,古代各个时期度量衡单位并不统一。如汉代,以斤、两、分、铢计量,1 斤相当于现代的 250 克。至宋代,以斤、两、钱、分、厘、毫剂量,1 斤相当于今天的 600 克。从 1979 年 1 月 1 日起,现代中药剂量改用标准单位"克",1 斤相当于 500 克。

1. 汉代　一斤＝250 克;一两＝15.625 克,一斤＝十六两;一分＝3.91 克,一两＝四分;一铢＝0.65 克,一两＝二十四铢。

2. 宋代　一斤＝600 克;一两＝37.5 克,一斤＝十六两;一钱＝3.75 克,一两＝十钱;一分＝0.375 克,一钱＝十分;一厘＝0.037 5 克,一分＝十厘;一毫＝0.003 75 克,一厘＝十毫。

3. 现代　一斤＝500 克,一两＝50 克,一钱＝5 克。如今"克"已成为现代中医最常用的剂量单位。

四、中医病案书写的意义与要求

1. 中医病案书写的意义　学习中医病案是积累临床经验的有效途径。如果你是一个初学者,从现代中医病案或明清相关文献开始学习,可能轻松得多。可惜的是,这些文献的英文版资源非常有限。学习古汉语知识会大大方便阅读,许多作者喜欢使用非常简洁的语言。学习病案时将临床表现、治疗方法和处方结合在一起,可以帮助您了解整个诊断和治疗过程。如果某些特定病案有其他医生的注释和评论,请不要错过。更多关注这些补充信息可能会帮助您从这些案例中提取更多有用的经验。说起来容易,实践难。但实践总能出真知。您阅读学习的中医病案越多,在日常诊疗实践中就可能做得越好。

2. 中医病案书写的具体要求 《中医病历书写基本规范》主要内容小结如下。

(1)中医病历书写通则

1)病历书写使用阿拉伯数字书写日期和时间,采用24小时制记录。

2)实习医务人员、试用期医务人员书写的病历,应经过本医疗机构注册的医务人员审阅、修改并签名。

3)病历应当使用蓝色或黑色墨水的钢笔书写,其他颜色的笔或圆珠笔书写病历是禁止且无效的。

(2)病历书写基本原则:客观、规范、专业、完整、准确、真实。

(3)门(急)诊病历书写内容及要求

1)门诊病历记录包括初诊病历记录和复诊病历记录。

2)病历首页应当包括患者姓名,性别,出生年、月、日,民族、婚姻状况、职业、住址、过敏史。

3)病历记录应当由接诊医师立即完成。

4)急诊病历应当记录患者去向。

5)急诊病历书写就诊时间应当具体到分钟。

(4)初诊病历记录

1)精确记录就诊时间、科别。

2)简洁的记录主诉(不超过20个汉字)。

3)记录现病史、既往史、中医四诊、阳性体征、必要的阴性体征和辅助检查结果。

4)记录诊断及治疗意见。

5)医生签名。

(5)复诊病历记录

1)每次就诊均需记录就诊时间、科别。

2)记录中医四诊、必要的体格检查和辅助检查结果。

3)进一步的诊断和治疗处理意见。

4)记录者或医生签名。

(6)急诊病历记录:急诊病历记录书写应当具体到分钟。

(7)现病史

1)本次疾病的发生,包括时间、地点、原因、症状、处理方法。

2）本次疾病的发展,包括医疗处理和症状体征的变化过程。

3）记录与主诉相关的具体表现。

4）补充中医的具体表现(以"十问歌"为基础,包括饮食、睡眠、二便等)。

5）近期阳性、必要的阴性体征以及中医四诊体征也需要详细记录。

（8）双重诊断系统

1）医师应同时记录西医诊断与中医诊断(包括中医病名和证候类型)。

2）西医诊断根据国际疾病分类(ICD)之 ICD - 10, ICD - 9 CM3;中医诊断根据国家标准《中医病证分类与代码》(TCD),如 GB95, GB97。

（9）诊疗原则

1）治疗计划应包含西医治疗和中医治疗。

2）当面对几种可选择的治疗方法时,医生应根据患者的整体情况选择最佳的治疗方法,最大限度地保护患者的权益。

3）用精确的专业术语记录。记录者应保证电子病历的逻辑性,手写病历应清晰可识别。

4）签名。

五、如何阅读医案

1. **顺读法**　依照医案书写的顺序,先读案语,了解症状、病因病机、诊断、治法以后,再看处方用药。此法适宜于读理法方药较严谨的实录式医案以及追忆式医案。

2. **逆读法**　即先看处方用药,以方测证,以药测证,然后再参考其案语。这种方法,对于一些案语简略,或仅列主症,或仅列主脉,或仅叙述病机而未载症状的医案最为适合。

3. **理读法**　即按照中医理论,从医案中记载的病名、病机、治法等来推测主症、主法,揣摩辨证论治、处方用药的思路与经验的方法。

前人医案的写法和现在的病历记载有所不同,主要是根据现有症状,抓住辨证立法的关键,虽然记载较简略,但有理论依据可循。

4. **比较法**　即通过两个以上的同类医案在主症、治法、方药上的相互比较,从而揭示作者辨证立法用药的主要经验与学术思想。

运用比较法的关键,是注意医案之间的可比性。按照中医的特点,一般可从病证、症状、治法、方药以及医家等方面进行比较和分类。

（1）同一位医家,同一种病证的医案比较,重在了解该病证的辨证论治规律。

（2）同一位医家,同一张方剂的医案比较,重在探讨该医家运用此方的经验。

（3）同一种病证,多位医家的医案比较,在于了解各家诊治此病的特色。

六、医案实例

头部病门

牙疼

天津王姓,年三十余,得牙疼病。

[病因] 商务劳心,又兼连日与友宴饮,遂得斯证。

[证候] 其牙疼甚剧,有碍饮食,夜不能寐,服一切治牙疼之药不效,已迁延二十余日矣。脉象其脉左部如常,而右部弦长,按之有力。

[诊断] 此阳明胃气不降也。

[处方] 生赭石(一两轧细) 怀牛膝(一两) 滑石(六钱) 甘草(一钱)

煎汤服。

[效果] 将药煎服一剂,牙疼立愈,俾按原方再服一剂以善其后。

[帮助] 方书治牙疼未见有用赭石、牛膝者,因愚曾病牙疼以二药治愈,后凡遇胃气不降致牙疼者,方中必用此二药。

该医案出自《医学衷中参西录》。

七、课后习题

(1) 中国第一位发明和使用病历的人是谁?他记录的内容包括什么?

(2) 请换算此古方的用药剂量:桂枝汤。

桂枝三两　　芍药三两　　生姜三两　　甘草二两　　大枣十二枚

该方出自汉代张仲景所著《伤寒论》。

参考文献

[1] 王阶.中医病历书写基本规范[M].北京:科学技术文献出版社,2010.

Chapter One

History and Development of TCM Records

No matter how smart you are or how good your memory is, keeping records is one of the most effective ways to note and recollect all the important information in detail. Especially if you're a doctor facing thousands of different patients, it is impossible to remember everything precisely. Hence, medical records are very important for every doctor to recall the patient encounter details and transmit information between colleagues.

1. Main History of Ancient TCM Record

The patient's medical record is a summary of patient's condition and about how the illness happened and developed, and was diagnosed and treated.

1.1 Early records (Since the Shang Dynasty to the Sui Dynasty) The earliest TCM records we know of today are inscriptions on animal bones and turtle shells of the Shang Dynasty (Figure 1-1). Among those precious ancient literature, records of 21 health related conditions were found. The well acknowledged earliest TCM records were "25 medical records" found in Shi Ji (also known as "Historical Records" written by Bian Que and Cang Gong dated to 2170 years ago in the Han Dynasty, Figure

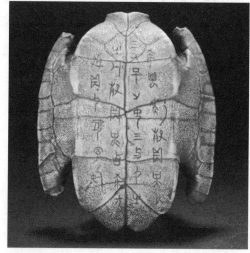

Figure 1 – 1   Inscriptions on animal bones and turtle shells of the Shang Dynasty
(Picture from California Asian Art Auction Gallery)

1 - 2). Several TCM records are also found in *Zhou Hou Bei Ji Fang* (Handbook of Prescriptions for Emergency written by Ge Hong in the Jin dynasty), and *Zhu Bing Yuan Hou Lun* ("General Treatise on the Cause and Symptoms of Diseases" by ChaoYuanfang from the Sui Dynasty). According to the current literature, the first person who invented and used medical records in China was Chun Yuyi, a famous doctor in the early Han Dynasty. He used to record the patient's name, address, symptoms, prescriptions, date of diagnosis and treatment, even the outcome (cure or death) of the patient. In the long run, Chun found that these records were of great benefit to help with diagnosis and treatment, so he named it "Zhen Ji".

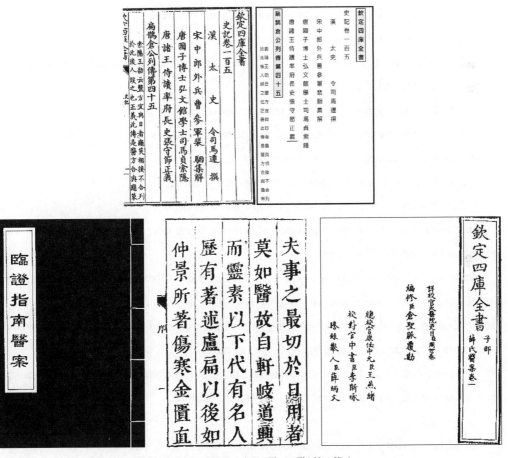

Figure 1 - 2　*Shi Ji* and *Lin Zheng Zhi Nan Yi An*
(Pictures from http：//ctext.org/library)

1.2　Boom stage(Since Tang Dynasty to Qing Dynasty)　Since the Tang and Song Dynasties, TCM records became more and more popular. The first monograph on TCM records in history is *Shang Han Jiu Shi Lun* ("90 discourses of Shanghan" by Xu Shuwei in the Song Dynasty). In the Ming and Qing Dynasties, doctors paid more and more attention to summarizing and publishing TCM records. Many famous masterpieces were found from this period, including the Dr Xue's *Medical Records* (by Xue Ji, Ming Dynasty) and *Lin Zheng Zhi Nan Yi An* (also known as "Medical Records to Guide Clinical Practice" by Ye Tianshi, Qing Dynasty). Nowadays, TCM doctors can still gain useful insights from those ancient literatures. In 1584, Wu Kun summarized a medical record format with 7 sections in his masterpiece *Mai Lun* (also known as "Analects of Diagnosis", Ming Dynasty). These sections included:

1.2.1　Time of encounter, patient's name and place of birth.

1.2.2　Findings of inspection and inquisition.

1.2.3　When did the conditions started, reasons for the illness, emotional states of patients, and related past history.

1.2.4　Primary diagnosis, therapies and outcomes.

1.2.5　If there were condition-related manifestations such as aversion to cold or heat and dietary preference and any time-related exacerbation.

1.2.6　Diagnosis, related reasons and therapeutic methods.

1.2.7　Prescriptions in details with principle and explanation.

He further emphasized the importance of doctor's signatures. His format has laid a solid foundation for modern TCM records.

Other works such as *the Ming Yi Lei An* ("Sorted Medical Records of Famous Doctors" by Jiang Guan, Qing Dynasty) and *Xu Ming Yi Lei An* ("Sequel of Sorted Medical Records of Famous Doctors" by Wei Zhixiu, Qing Dynasty) are outstanding literatures on TCM record, which are widely read and studied by TCM doctors today.

However, due to the limit of the dynasties, those monographs were all results of personal practice, and no standardized format could be widely followed.

2. Main History of Western Medicine (WM) Record

Prior to 1900, there was no standard format for keeping medical records in WM history. In fact, many doctors did not even touch their patients other than to check the pulse. Medicine and Astrology were cognate disciplines. However, unlike astrologers, medical practitioners had no need to work with a pen in hand. They diagnose the disease from the patient's complexion, urine and other excretions. There was no so much data to be recorded. Medical practitioners seem to have begun keeping written records much later than the astrologers, and these records are more diverse in nature. They fall into roughly three categories. The most rudimentary records were lists of the names of clients and their payments for treatments or prescriptions. These are account books, and need to be understood alongside the broader trends of record keeping which developed in late medieval Europe. In Europe, narratives of cures were recorded in ancient Greek medical record and this practice was widely used in the fourteenth and fifteenth centuries. Some of these recorded advice were about diet and recipes to patients; others were framed as testimonials of

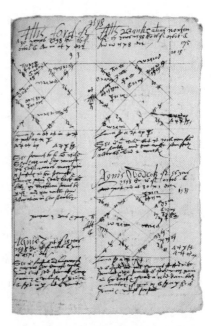

Figure 1 – 3   The Casebooks of Simon Foreman and Richard Napier
Picture from papyrus to the electronic tablet: a brief history of the clinical medical record with lessons for the digital age.

successful or remarkable cures, autopsies or lessons for surgeons. These elements were expanded and multiplied in the sixteenth century. As part of this trend, medical practitioners began keeping collections of case summaries that they called "observations" (Figure 1 – 3). In the following decades "case records" began to be kept in hospitals, signaling the promotion of systematic and objective medical practices.

Examples of these publications include Forman's and Napier's casebooks that pre-date modern medical records.

3. The Development of The Modern TCM Record

Following the foundation of the People's Republic of China, many TCM hospitals were founded. However, the medical records kept within these establishments were all made in so-called WM format. In 1982, the China Association of Chinese Medicine (CACM) drafted the first version of the "Format and Requirements for TCM Records". After piloting of this draft recommendation, revisions have since been made. In 1988, the State Administration of TCM

（SATCM） asked the CACM to finalized this national standard with nation-wide experts consultation and amendment. In 1991, the "*Regulation on TCM Records*" was officially released and put into practice. In 2002, The "*Regulation on the Handling of Medical Accidents*" was passed into legislation and put into clinical practice. As a supplement of the national legal "*Regulation on Records of TCM*", the WM and TCM Integrative Trial was officially released.

The current regulation on keeping TCM records is the 2010 version, which was drafted by the requirements from the national health and family planning commission （NHFPC） and the state administration of TCM （SATCM）. This has been implemented since July 1, 2002 and revised in 2010. The requirement includes four sections: a. Basic requirement, b. Clinic （emergency） record requirements and writing content, c. Inpatient medical record writing content and requirements, and d. Print medical record requirements. For inpatients, the main records have different requirements in different countries and include items such as the admission note （24 hours）, the initial progress note （8 hours）, the record of the first round （48 hours）, the record of the attending daily round, progress notes, etc. Especially for history of present illness, in China, besides the occurrence and the development of disease, the procedure of diagnosis and treatment prior to admission and the present manifestation of the illness, there should be TCM cause, pathogenesis, manifestation （based on the Ten Question Song, appetite, sleep quality, stool and urine）, and treatment. Regarding diagnosis, the double diagnosis systems current practiced in China includes WM diagnosis and TCM diagnosis. Regarding the treatment principle and strategy, the treatment should also include both WM and TCM options.

Note: History of Standardization on the Dose Unit in TCM

The dosage of TCM in prescriptions is generally guided by the latest edition of the Pharmacopoeia of the People's Republic of China and is determined according to the nature of drugs, preparations, compatibility, age, constitution, illness of patients and seasonal changes. At present, the dosage of TCM is gradually converted from ancient classics criteria and combined with long-term clinical practice. In different dynasties, the dosages of medicine were determined by different units. For example: in the Han Dynasty, this was measured by Jin,

Liang, Fen and Zhu measuring units. At that time, 1 Jin was equivalent to about 250 g today. In the Song Dynasty, it was measured using Jin, Liang, Qian, Fen, Li and Hao measuring units. But at this time 1 Jin was about 600 g today. Since January 1, 1979, the standard dose unit of modern Chinese medicine has been changed to gram （g）, and 1 Jin equals to 500 g today.

Han Dynasty:

1 Jin（斤） 250 g

1 Liang（两） 15.625 g   1 Jin = 16 Liang

1 Fen(分) 3.91 g   1 Liang = 4 Fen

1 Zhu(铢) 0.65   1 Liang = 24 Zhu

Song Dynasty:

1 Jin(斤) 600 g

1 Liang(两) = 37.5 g   1 Jin = 16 Liang

1 Qian(钱) = 3.75 g   1 Liang = 10 Qian

1 Fen(分) = 0.375 g   1 Qian = 10 Fen

1 Li (厘) = 0.037 5 g   1 Fen = 10 Li

1 Hao(毫) = 0.003 75 g   1 Li = 10 Hao

Current unit system:

1 Jin(斤) = 500 g

1 Liang(两) = 50 g

1 Qian(钱) = 5 g

Now gram(g, 克) is the most commonly used unit for current dosage of TCM

4. Significance and Requirement of TCM record

4.1   Significance   Studying TCM records is an efficient way to improve your clinical experience. If you are a beginner, starting with the contemporary medical records or the related literatures from Ming and Qing Dynasties could be much easier. Unfortunately, there are very limited resources of English versions of these books. Learning some ancient Chinese would significantly facilitate your reading. Many authors preferred to use very concise language. Combining the documentation of clinical manifestation, therapeutic methods and prescriptions together, may help you in understanding the whole process of diagnosis and treatment. Do not ignore any annotations and comments from other doctors on a particular case summary. Paying more attention to this supplementary information may help you extract more useful experience and great ideas from these cases. This is much easier said than done, but practice always makes perfect. The more you read and learn from TCM records, the better you can apply these principles in your daily practice.

4.2   Requirement   The summary of "Regulation on records of TCM":

4.2.1   Basic requirement of medical record in summary

4.2.1.1   Medical record writing uses Arabic numerals to write the date and time, with 24-hour format.

4.2.1.2   The records written by interns, medical staffs in probation period should be reviewed, modified and signed by the qualified medical personnel.

4.2.1.3   Use blue or black ink pen to write, other color pen or ball-pen is forbidden and invalid.

4.2.2   Principle of Medical Records   objective, normative, professional, complete, accurate, authentic.

4.2.3   Clinic (emergency) record requirements and writing content

4.2.3.1   Clinical record includes initial visit and subsequence visit.

4.2.3.2   Record's homepage includes: name, gender, birthday, ethnic, marital status, occupation, address and allergy history.

4.2.3.3   Record should be finished by the doctors in charge at once.

4.2.3.4   In an emergency situation, where the patient is transferred to should be recorded.

4.2.3.5   The arrival time of emergency medical record should be specific to the minute.

4.2.4   Initial visit

4.2.4.1   Time and department should be precisely recorded.

4.2.4.2   Write down the chief complaint in a concise way (the number of Chinese characters are usually limited to 20).

4.2.4.3   Record history of present illness, past history, TCM "four diagnosis" findings, positive and necessary negative signs and auxiliary examination results.

4.2.4.4   Record the diagnosis and related treatments advice.

4.2.4.5   Last but not least, the signature of recorder and/or doctor.

4.2.5   Subsequent visits

4.2.5.1   Time and department should be recorded every time.

4.2.5.2   Record TCM "four diagnosis", the necessary physical examination and auxiliary examination results after last visit.

4.2.5.3   Make further diagnosis, treatment, disposal and record these.

4.2.5.4   Signature of recorder and/or doctor.

4.2.6   Emergency record   Emergency medical record writing time should be specific to minutes.

4.2.7   History of present illness

4.2.7.1   The occurrence of disease includes: time, place, reason, symptom and disposal.

4.2.7.2   The development of disease contains the medical disposal and the change process of signs and symptoms.

4.2.7.3   Record the present manifestation relevant to the chief complaint in detail.

4.2.7.4   Supplement the specific present manifestation of TCM (based on ten question song, appetite, sleep quality, stool and urine).

4.2.7.5   Present positive and necessary negative signs and specific TCM four diagnosis signs should be obtained and written down as well.

4.2.8 Double diagnosis systems

4.2.8.1 In the part, doctor should record both WM diagnosis and TCM diagnosis (with both TCM disease and pattern).

4.2.8.2 Refer to the standard of WM codes from ICD − 10, ICD − 9 CM3(procedure) and TCM codes from TCD(GB95, GB97).

4.2.9 Treatment principle and strategy

4.2.9.1 Therapeutic plan for patient includes both WM and TCM ways.

4.2.9.2 When facing several optional ways, doctor should choose the treatment to maximize benefits of patient according to his overall condition.

4.2.9.3 Write it down with accurate terms and wording. The recorder should ensure the electronic record in a logic way and if the record has been done in handwriting, the whole record should be recognizable.

4.2.9.4 Signature.

5. How To Read TCM Record

5.1 Forward reading

5.1.1 First read the comments.

5.1.2 Then understand the symptoms, pathology, diagnosis and treatment.

5.1.3 Finally read the prescription.

Forward reading is generally used on veritable record and reminiscing record.

5.2 Reverse (backwards) reading
Read the medication prescribed first, deduce the pattern of disease from the formula, deduce the pattern from the herbs, then refer to the comments. This method is best suited for cases where the comment is abbreviated, or there is only the main symptoms or only the main pulse, or the case of pathogen being recorded without symptom description.

5.3 Understand reading

5.3.1 To speculate the main pattern, main treatments, pattern differentiation and prescription thinking, from ancient medical records' disease name, pathogenesis and treatment.

5.3.2 Ancient record's writing method, which is based on symptom and the key of differentiation and treating principle, is different from modern record. Though it was recorded simply, there are theoretical basis.

5.4 Comparison method

5.4.1 Compare the main pattern, treatment, and prescription, to reveal the main syndrome differentiation and treatment selection experience and academic thought through two or more similar cases.

The key to use the comparison method, is to pay attention to the comparability between records. Generally from the disease pattern, symptom, treatment, and the formulas used on can base on the acknowledgement and classification by comparison. Here are some concrete methods below:

5.4.2 Compare all the records about the same kind of disease from the same doctor to understand the rule of syndrome differentiation and treatment.

5.4.3 Compare the records with the same formula from the same doctor to discuss the doctor's experience in applying the formula.

5.4.4 Compare the records about the same disease from various doctors to understand the features on the diagnosis and treatment from them.

6. Case Report

Facial Disease Part

Odontalgia

Mr. Wang, who was in his thirties, lived in Tianjin, presented with a toothache.

Pathogeny: Busy business and uncontrolled party with drinking without restraint.

Syndrome: A serious toothache for more than 20 days affecting appetite and causing insomnia. Medication did not have a good curative effect.

Pulse Condition: Normal pulse on the left hand, wiry, powerful and long on the other.

Diagnosis: Undescending of Yangming gastric qi

Prescription: Sheng Zheshi (1 ounce, powder-like)

Huai Niuxi(1 ounce)

Huashi(0.6 ounce)

Gancao(0.1 ounce)

Decocted in water

Curative Effect: Quickly recovered after a dose, and continue with one more dose to consolidate efficacy.

Tips: In medical records before, no one had used Haematitum and Achyranthes bidentate for the treatment of toothache, but after I cured my own toothache by these two herbs accidently, I adopted these in my practice to manage toothache.

This medical record is from *the Records of Traditional Chinese and Western Medicine in Combination*.

One hopes that you enjoy a wonderful journey when reading this textbook and become an expert in both making and studying TCM records. The book is a treasure house of information that could potentially be a powerful weapon in treating diseases.

7. Homework

Homework 1　Who was the first person in China to invent and use medical records? What did he record?

Homework 2　Please convert the dosage of this ancient prescription comes from *the Shanghan Lun* by Zhang Zhongjing in the Han Dynasty. Guizhi Tang:

Guizhi 3 liang

Shaoyao 3 liang

Shengjiang 3 liang

Gancao 2 liang

Dazao 12 mei

References

[1] Wang J. Regulation on records of TCM[M]. Beijing: Scientific and Technical Documentation, 2010.

第二章 医学写作与"诚信"

医学写作是所有领域的研究者传播其研究新的创意、方法和结果的重要手段。研究者通过期刊、网络等平台交流和分享自身在其专业领域的研究成果，不断推动该学科的创新发展。随着世界各国科研建设投入的增加，全球范围内的论文发表数量也呈现较快增长态势。

"诚信"是人类社会形成与发展中构建人与人和谐关系的纽带和桥梁。论文写作中的"诚信"是研究者职业道德素养的体现，是研究成果真实呈现的重要保障，是各学科实现创新发展的重要动力。

随着中医药科学化、标准化的发展以及中医药研究体系的建立，中医药研究的数量和质量得到较快的增长和提高。中医药研究已经成为中医药发展与创新的时代符号。作为中医药研究的重要组成部分，中医药论文写作不仅有利于中医药研究成果的分享，更有利于中医药的不断创新和推广。中医药论文写作中的"诚信"建设，是推动中医药正确、健康发展的重要保证。

一、"诚信"的概念

诚信，英文"integrity"，起源于拉丁语"integer"，原意为"完整，一体"，后延伸为人的品格的"完整"，也就是"诚信，真诚"。"诚信"在中国拥有悠久的历史，起初"诚"与"信"并未合并使用，在《逸周书》中则第一次把二者合并使用"成年不尝，信诚匡助，以辅殖材"。孟子说："诚者，天之道也，诚者，人之道也。"《中庸》说："诚者，天之道，诚之者，人之道。""诚信"在中国古代被视为大自然的规律，被视为人的规律。现代，"诚信"指遵守承诺、言行一致、态度真诚。

学术诚信，英文"academic integrity"，是在学术领域内根据学术发展的要求和规律而形成的、以研究者为对象的诚信规范。学术诚信的形成与优化是学术发展的必然结果。目前，随着人们诚信意识的不断提高,世界各地把"学术诚信"放在了高等教育中学生培养的重要环节,许多高校、科研院所相继发布了关于"学术诚信"的相关要求。

论文写作诚信是诚信的重要组成部分,要求作者在写用于发表的论文时必须以事实为依据,诚实、完整地呈现研究的相关内容和创新点。目前,国内外许多杂志均颁布了其论文写作的诚信要求,同时也引入了论文写作诚信辨别与查找的相关工具。

二、医学论文写作中的"不端"

在很多国家和地区,医学论文的发表与研究者职称晋升有直接联系,这种现状导致了部分学者盲目追求论文发表数量,而导致不符合"诚信"的"不端"行为出现。一般而言,在论文写作中的"不端"行为主要为"剽窃"和"造假"两种。

(一) 剽窃

"剽窃"是指在论文写作过程中,作者有意或无意地把其他作者文章中的数据、图表以及创意占为己有,且不添加文献索引说明。"剽窃"是医学论文写作中最常见的"不端"现象,其按照"剽窃"的内容来源分为"一般剽窃"和"自我剽窃"。

1. 一般剽窃

(1) 概念与简介:"一般剽窃"是指作者完全复制原作者的语句、段落,且无文献索引说明或无获得授权。常见现象为作者把不同作者的文章通过剪切和拼接,或剪切原作者文章的研究数据、图表等信息,组合成一篇自己的新论文署名并发表。

(2)"一般剽窃"的危害

1) 缺乏对原作者的尊重:"一般剽窃"的主要特点是把其他作者的研究结果、数据、图表等不加引用地占为己有。原作者通过科学的实验研究设计和实验过程以及严谨的逻辑论证最终编写了具有创新性、科学性的论文。每一篇论文从创意到数据、信息、结论以及文字的编纂都是原作者思想和智慧的载体,是原作者不辞辛苦努力劳动的成果。不加引用地占据他人论文成果与信息是对他人劳动成果的侵犯,是对原作者极大的不尊重。

2) 危害自身:"一般剽窃"不仅不尊重原作者的智慧成果,也对剽窃者本身产生一定的直接危害。一方面,"一般剽窃"将使作者失信于人。每一篇论文都是自己"创新"的逻辑论证,因此论文的发表是共享学术创新的重要方面。"一般剽窃"所产生的论文既缺乏"新创意",同时也缺乏严谨的逻辑论证,只是文字的堆砌,这必将塑造一个消极的科研形象。同时,随着各杂志社加大对"剽窃"行为的管控,"一般剽窃"将使杂志社失去对作者的信任,对其今后论文的发表产生直接的影响。另一方面,"一般剽窃"将阻碍作者的职称发展。已发表论文的数量是大部分学术机构考量学者科研成绩的重要指标,学者在其领域内的论文发表数量直接影响职称的晋升。为提高科研论文发表的质量,"一般剽窃"逐渐被各大学术机构纳入"学术不端"行为,且给予极高的重视。各大机构对"一般剽窃"等"学术不端"行为进行了严格的管控,其中"一票否决"最具有代表性。如果作者从事"一般剽窃"被记录在案,将极大地影响其在学术圈内的职称评定和晋升。

3）资源浪费：论文既是劳动成果,也是科研再创新的优良资源。已发表的论文是新的科研研究设计、开展以及逻辑论证的重要基础。随着各个国家地区加大推动科研发展的力度,不同语言、不同国家的论文发表成为全球科研创新交流的重要形式。论文已经成为全球各领域不断创新发展的重要资源。然而,"一般剽窃"虽然增加了论文的数量,但是缺乏新创意和逻辑论证,质量较低。"一般剽窃"是对他人研究成果的再重复,缺乏其应有的科研理论价值,是科研资源的重大浪费。

4）不利于学科创新性发展：前期研究是学科创新发展的重要基础。因此,学科的创新发展不仅需要庞大的论文数量支撑,更需要高质量的论文品质保证。剽窃和重复他人的科研成果造成了低质量的学术论文,对于学科创新发展不具备任何价值和意义。同时,如果作者不当地重复或断章取义、扭曲原作者的真实观点将对该学科的创新发展带来极大的不利影响。

（3）如何避免"一般剽窃"

1）以"自己的创意"为中心。"一般剽窃"的主要特点是把他人研究创意、方法等占为己有。任何研究的设计与开展必须基于主要研究者新的创意。论文写作是通过详细阐述研究过程实现"自我创意"的过程。在创意实现的过程中,文献的引用能够有效地支撑"自己的创意"。因此,在论文写作之前,必须首先明确自己的创意和已有文献所描述的创意。在写作过程中,必须以"自己的创意"为中心,以实验数据和已有文献为辅助,全面地证明"自己的创意"的可行性。清晰地辨别"自己的创意"与"已有文献的创意"是避免"一般剽窃"的前提。

2）标明文献引用索引。任何文章的立论必须以前人研究成果为基础。引用文献中其他作者的创意、数据或其他信息是论文写作中不可缺少的环节。标明文献引用索引是辨别是否"剽窃"的重要标准。因此,在论文写作中,必须清晰地、准确地注明文献索引和来源。① 何时需要索引：一方面,当我们从外部资源（指除了与文章相关的研究之外）中搜寻时,无论我们整段引用或是部分引用,都必须注明索引。另一方面,当我们用自己的语言重新组织外部资源信息时,也需要注明外部资源的来源。② 如何使用索引：一般情况下,网络URL或日期能够充分表达外部资源的来源信息;在重新组织语言表达外部资源信息时,我们需要注明"adapted from"或"based on",以使读者辨别外来资源的信息;咨询即将投递的杂志,一般杂志都有其独特的要求。

(4) 中医写作中的合理引用:引用中医经典和古籍中的理论不属于剽窃的范畴。作者可以通过引用经典来阐述自己的观点。但需要注意的是,引用时应明确标注出处和作者名。

2. 自我剽窃 "自我剽窃"一般指作者在新的文章中,出现与该作者已发表文章重复、再利用的现象。除了逐字逐段的文本外,在不同的地方出版相同的论文(有时也称为"重复出版物")也可称之为"自我剽窃"。简而言之,自我剽窃是试图将以前发表过的任何文本、论文或研究成果,将其看作是全新的重复出版。萨拉米饼切片式和文字再利用都是自我剽窃的常见形式。

(1) 一稿多投

1) 概念与简介:"一稿多投",有时称"重复出版",一篇文章投递至两个及以上的杂志。"一稿多投"一定程度上能够增加作者论文发表的数量,但是属于"不端"行为,直接影响其职业发展。然而,"重合"并不是判定"一稿多投"的唯一衡量要素。以下情形虽然存在"重合",但是并不被认为是"一稿多投"。① 转换语言。一些学者为扩大其研究的影响,同时用多种语言发表至不同期刊中,或把已发表的文章转换成另一种语言发表至相应的区域中。目前,许多杂志允许作者通过语言转换发送至不同的期刊中,且不被视为重复发表。② 投递至截然不同领域的期刊中。随着各学科的不断交叉,部分研究的范围也存在一定的跨领域现象。因此,有些学者把同一篇文章投递至截然不同的学科领域,以拓展其研究在不同领域的影响力。每一个期刊都有其特有的或针对性的阅读群体,如化学期刊主要针对化学领域学者,医药期刊主要针对医药学者。这种行为并不会导致读者资源搜索的交叉,因此不属于"重复出版"。

2) "一稿多投"的危害:① 延缓论文的出版效率。论文在期刊的出版是一个过程,一般包括初审、终审与出版三个阶段。"一稿多投"至同一期刊或不同期刊,导致了一篇论文的重复审核,增加了论文审核和编辑的工作量。通常,一篇论文只能一次投递至一个杂志。如果作者"一稿多投",在论文审核编辑过程中不得不花费更多的精力于查找论文的重复投递,极大地延缓了论文出版、发表的效率。② 浪费资源。"一稿多投"使一篇论文不合理地占用杂志的版面资源,造成版面资源的极大浪费。每一个期刊的版面资源是有限的,期刊在编辑过程中也一直追求着版面资源的最大利用。"一稿多投"导致一篇论文同时占用其他期刊的版面资源,不利于版面资源的价值利用最大化。

3) 如何避免"一稿多投":① 作者应根据与杂志签订的投递协议,一篇手稿投递至一个杂志。② 如果投递正在审议的论文至其他杂志,应征得合作杂志的同意。③ 作者在涉及语言转换或投递不同领域期刊时,提前咨询相关刊物并详细说明已投情况,征询期刊意见,确定不属于"一稿多投"。④ 如果确定投递另一本杂志,应通知首杂志,申请撤回稿件,并获得首杂志稿件撤回证明。在重新投递论文至另一本杂志时,应随附稿件撤回证明。⑤ 如果写了两篇相似的论文,准备投递至两个不同的杂志,应向两家杂志披露两篇论文的细节,并提交另一副本。

（2）萨拉米饼切片式

1）概念及简介:"萨拉米饼切片式",英文"Salami-slicing",是指作者以同一个研究为基础,把实验研究的成果分成若干部分写作、发表的"不端"行为。其与"重复出版"的本质区别是不存在文献"重合"。其被分割的若干论文内容的假设、方法和出版杂志均相同。Salami-slicing 能够提高作者的论文数量,但是降低了每篇论文的质量,对于研究成果的分享交流产生了非常大的消极影响。

2）"萨拉米饼切片式"的危害: ① 降低论文质量。Salami-slicing 把同一研究成果切割成多部分分别发表于杂志,虽然能够提高论文的数量,但是破坏了科研研究成果的完整性,降低了论文的质量。一般而言,一个科研项目只围绕一个新创意,或只解决一个新问题。研究者围绕创意和问题在前期研究的基础上进行科学的设计和严谨的实验过程,最终论证新创意的合理性或提供具有可行性的新问题解决方法。Salami-slicing 把一个完整的科研过程和科研成果分割成若干部分,严重破坏了科研创新和科研体系的完整性,导致发表论文的分析和论证过于表浅,缺乏深度,严重降低论文的质量。② 缩减研究成果影响力,不利于科研创新。Salami-slicing 降低了论文的质量,为其影响力的扩展带来不利影响。Salami-slicing 所发表的论文是研究成果的分割,虽然每一篇论文均进行了一定的讨论,但是较之完整的论文讨论较为表浅。另外,被分割成多篇的论文,其在分析讨论中,缺乏或弱化了整个研究全局角度的分析讨论。读者在搜索相关文献时,存在很大的遗漏,不能完全领悟该研究的理论成果和意义。从某种意义上来讲 Salami-slicing 削弱了研究成果的影响力。

3）如何避免"萨拉米饼切片式":Salami-slicing 严重降低了研究论文的质量。该"不端"行为是研究者的主观行为。因此避免该"不端"行为的主要方式是研究者正确地认识到 Salami-slicing 的危害,从自身做起,杜绝 Salami-slicing 的发生。作者在写作前应详细罗列本研究的目的、内容和细节,归类排列并详细地在同一篇论文之中加以体现。

4）中医写作中的"萨拉米饼切片式":Salami-slicing 是中医写作中最常见的"不端"行为。中医诊断有寒热、虚实、阴阳之分。一疾病常包含多个证型。在进行中医相关研究时,同一疾病,不同证候,其给药和处理方式各不相同,得到的结论也会有所差异。而一些作者会根据其结果的多样性进行分割,从而增加论文的发表数量。这是不可取的。因此,作为中医学研究者,我们应将一项研究所得的多种结论发表在一篇论文中,从而避免 Salami-slicing 的"不端"行为。

（3）文字再利用

1）概念及介绍:"文字再利用"是指论文中多次出现作者自身已发表的论文中的句子或

段落。已发表论文中的句子和段落与现论文句子和段落的"重合程度"被视为判定"文字再利用不端行为"的重要标尺。但是,"重合程度"是一个范围尺度,目前,仍然没有"文字再利用"的重合度判定的共识,不同杂志的范围要求不尽相同。

在论文发表中,以下情形不属于"文字再利用"的"不端行为":① 引用部门规章(如伦理审查申请、动物管理中心文件等)或用来描述研究的目的、背景、预期结果等内容的研究内部文件。② 引用用于传播的且不具有版权的宣传资料或会议材料。

2)"文字再利用"的危害:① 干扰读者。读者通常会关注新发表论文中的新观点。作者"文字再利用"会使旧的观点出现在新的论文中,导致读者对于新旧观点的混淆,不利于读者从新发表的论文中筛选信息。② 发表的资源浪费。"文字再利用"会使编辑重复审核已发表的内容,增加了重复工作量,且违背了论文发表的目的和原则,占用了有限的杂志版面。

3)如何避免"文字再利用":① 尽量不要复制过多的内容。为了避免重复出版,我们不应该从以前发表的论文中复制更多的内容。② 不要从已发表文章中直接复制内容。已发表的文章虽然公布的作者为作者本人,但是其在期刊发表时已经把文章引用权转交于期刊,因此直接复制已发表文章的部分内容属于侵权和"不端"行为。③ 未经杂志许可,不得向媒体、公司或其他机构提供有关未发表论文的初步报告。④ 不要从原有文章中过多地引用句子,在少量引用时需注明索引和来源。⑤ 如果存在"重合",应及时告知杂志社,并提交"重合"论文的详细信息,以便于杂志社合理判定是否为"重复出版"。

(二)造假

1. 概念及介绍 "造假"是指作者在论文写作中,违背实验实际结果的行为。伯克利大学定义"造假"为"在任何学术活动中,编造数据、信息和文献引用的行为"。伪造实验数据、表格以及参考文献是最常见的论文写作"造假"。论文造假不仅违背了客观、真实、科学的实验精神,同时也有极大可能为学科发展和社会建设带来严重的危害。

2."造假"的危害

(1)自身信誉。"造假"对作者的信誉造成严重的影响。"造假"与"剽窃"不同,其"不端"的负面影响更为严重。在医学研究中,"造假"可能对公众的健康造成严重危害。因此,许多机构对于"造假"出台了更为严厉的处罚条例。学术造假不仅会毁掉作者在学术领域的信誉,同时他还需要承担相应的法律责任。

(2)不利于学科建设与创新发展。科学研究的目的是以加强创新和发展为原则。对于一个创新的科学研究,关于它的设计、实验、分析都将以作者相关研究为基础。医学研究领域的学术造假将会为该实验后续的研究提供错误的导向,导致背离相关学科研究的发展方向,阻碍了其正确地良好发展。

（3）危害公众健康。医学研究的主要目的是通过科学的实验设计来探索某疾病关于病因学、发病机制、治疗等方面的新发现。通过对实验的详细描述，以及对其研究结果合理分析，为疾病治疗提供新的方向，为公众健康提供正确的指南。医务工作者常常将其作为对疾病诊断、治疗的重要参考，根据指南上最新、最有效的治疗方案来诊疗患者，从而提高治愈率。对于研究目的、样本量的大小、实验方法、实验结果的造假，不仅会阻碍学科的创新与发展，还将会严重误导临床诊疗工作，甚而危害公众健康。

3. 如何避免"造假"

（1）及时、准确地记录实验数据、实验结果。及时、客观记录是保证实验数据真实反映实验情况的重要措施。研究者在实验过程中，应详细记录每一个实验的细节，及时总结和评估实验的阶段性成果。

（2）实验过程中的细微异常，应及时分析原因，不可随意忽略。

（3）文献引用时，应保证足够的时间搜集和整理参考文献。

（4）了解杂志对参考文献引用格式的要求。

（5）仔细检查已完成的文件，并附上检查报告。

三、引用

引用是写作过程中所必须的。当读者在阅读论文时，一些引用的观点可以为其阅读原始文献提供参考。一般而言，参考文献常包含作者名、文献题目、杂志名、出版日期和页码。罗列参考文献是避免"剽窃"的重要方式。

1. 参考文献的必要性

（1）方便读者追溯和讨论原始文献论点的正确性。这是参考文献的一个重要的作用。读者在阅读文献的过程中常常需要追溯原始文献，去查找他们感兴趣的资料。参考文献可以帮助读者定位相关文献，以便收集相应的资料。另外，读者在阅读过程中需要通过原始数据来再次判定原先观点的合理性和正确性。

（2）论证作者的观点。在论文中阐述自己的观点时可以通过引用他人的文献来支撑自己的论点。适当引用文献可以为自己的论点提供论据。此外，通过引用可以将自己的论点与他人的观点进行比较，阐述自身观点的创新性和讨论价值。

2. 什么时候需要罗列参考文献   只要对他人的观点进行了引用，我们就应该将其写入参考文献中。具体需要罗列参考文献的情况如下。

（1）引用他人的词句。

（2）复述他人的观点。

（3）引用他人的论点。

（4）参考他人的研究方法。

（5）与自己的论点有较大不同的观点。

3. 如何引用避免"不端"行为 罗列参考文献是唯一规避"不端"行为的方式。在书写参考文献的过程中，作者不仅需要关注引用文献的格式，还应通过一些方法避免"不端"。以下提供一些可以规避"不端"的有效方法。

（1）复述资料，避免直接引用。在文献引用的过程中，自己组织语言来复述是降低重复率的常用方法。复述的方法总结如下：改变句子结构；用同义词进行替换；改变书写的语气；改变措辞；改变部分论点。

（2）直接引用，并做好标注。

四、课后推荐阅读

Duplicate Publication, Office of Research Integrity（DHHS）.

五、课后习题

（1）说说论文写作"不端"行为的概念及预防措施。

（2）结合自身经历，谈谈自己对论文写作"不端"的看法。

参考文献

[1] 宾夕法尼亚大学.避免抄袭：当有疑问时，引用[EB/OL].[2017-04-13]. http://www.upenn.edu/academicintegrity/ai_citingsources.html.

[2] 美国卫生与人类服务部.重复出版[EB/OL].[2017-04-07]. http://ori.hhs.gov/plagiarism-14.

[3] 意得辑.重复出版与一稿多投[EB/OL].[2017-04-14]. http://www.editage.com/insights/duplicate-publications-and-simultaneous-submissions.

[4] 处理.文字再利用[EB/OL].[2017-04-18]. https://publicationethics.org/files/Web_A29298_COPE_Text_Recycling.

[5] 伯克利城市学院.什么是学术造假？[EB/OL].[2017-04-15]. http://www.berkeleycitycollege.edu/wp/de/what-is-academic-dishonesty.

[6] 得克萨斯大学达拉斯分校.学术造假[EB/OL].[2017-04-14]. http://www.utdallas.edu/conduct/dishonesty.

Chapter Two

Integrity in Medical Writing for Publication

Medical writing is a pivotal way for researchers to share their new ideas, new methods and new results. A number of papers may be published to explore an unknown academic field or to amplify on prevalent knowledge.

Honesty and integrity are important essential attributes to academic writing. With integrity, the articles published not only increase quantity, but enhance quality. Integrity assures the development of the innovation of medicine.

The core objective of TCM writing for publication is to share the consequence of the research. With the development of TCM studies, publications have been an effective and efficient route to communicate the achievements of the various facets of TCM research. The quantity and quality of TCM innovation have been promoted by the sharing of the ideas, methods and conclusions of research that have been published in journals. TCM writing, a carrier of the information and data from the research, is closely related to the TCM sharing, and makes important contributions to the development of TCM.

1. About Integrity and Academic Integrity

"Integrity", origins from the Latin adjective "integer", means complying with the honesty, truthfulness or accuracy of one's action. Some dictionaries define it as being honest and having strong moral principles. In China, integrity has been an important social morality for thousands of years. Mencius views integrity as one of the rules of nature. Integrity has always been a core concept of human society.

Academic integrity refers to the application of integrity values in the academic field. It demands the staff in the academic world to act with integrity. With the brand of the integrity concept, academic integrity has been an important part of education in colleges and universities. Almost all of the universities have developed rules about the academic meaning of integrity.

Integrity in medical writing is one facet of academic integrity, referring to the importance that the author must be honest in his reporting of his findings and should not resort to fraud in the publication. Integrity in medical writing further requires accurate citation of any material previously generated by other people. Such action would result in plagarism.

2. Misconduct in Medical Writing

Academic publications reflect with the author's academic grading. This can be a stimulus to academic misconduct by promoting plagiarism and fabrication of results to gain academic points.

2.1 Plagiarism　　Plagiarism is regarded as the most frequently occurring form of dishonesty in medical research writing. This is considered to have taken place when authors represent other authors' work as their own, including the unreferenced use of another author's ideas, interpretations or data. Plagiarism consists of two forms: common form and self-plagiarism form.

2.1.1　Common form of plagiarism

2.1.1.1　Introduction: The common form of plagiarism occurs when the author copies another author's work word-by-word, for example, use another author's tables or figures without acknowledging the source and obtaining permission for use, cut and paste sentences or paragraphs and piece them together as one's own, and use other author's data or conclusions without citing the reference.

2.1.1.2　Why should we avoid plagiarism

2.1.1.2.1　Lack of respects to original author: The main common form of plagiarism is passing on other author's information (the results, data and figures from other journals written by other authors) as one's own. The original author would have explored and proved the idea by the rigorous design and practice of the research carried out. The idea, data, conclusion and editing are an achievement of that author's labor. Using that information without acknowledgement fails to show respect to the work carried out by the original author.

2.1.1.2.2　Harmful to the author him/herself: Another common form of plagiarism is harmful to the author him/herself. This form of plagiarism results in dishonesty to others. An academic paper is an opportunity to prove an idea by using logistical scientifically approved methods. Plagiarized publications are deplete of new ideas or in the logic argument. This affects the readers and the scientific community adversely. With the control of the journals to the common form of plagiarism, this style of plagiarism is considered to lose the credit of the journals. On the other hand, common form would strike out the grading of the academic. The number of papers published by a researcher is often related to the academic standing. Many journals and academic institutions have grasped control of this form of plagiarism, where the model "One vote veto" is inbuilt. If this type of plagiarism is registered and reported, the opportunity to grade an academic would be deprived by the academic institutions.

2.1.1.2.3　Waste of the source of journal: Not only the publication of a paper is an achievement in itself, but also it is a source that could be used in propagating future research. Papers published in the journals carry all of the details and results produced in the research, which build the foundation for the next research project. Publications have been potential sources that push academic innovation. However, plagiarized papers lack new ideas and new results. They are furthermore considered as a waste of journal resources.

2.1.1.2.4　Hinder to the innovative development of the subject.　Early stage researches are the foundation of a new innovation if founded on high quality papers. Plagiarism produces papers of low quality, which hinders innovation. In addition, the plagiarizing author would be distorting the reality and the truth that should be reflected in the research. So, the plagiarism is of no benefit to academic innovation.

2.1.1.3　How can one avoid plagiarism

2.1.1.3.1　This concept is central to this article. The common form of plagiarism is an intentional dishonesty in medical writing. The feature of the common plagiarism is to assume other authors' work and pass it on as one's own. So, the author should clearly identify the ideas which are his/her and those ideas that belong to others. Every academic paper published should articulate the author's finding and ideas. The references and the sources that we have acknowledgment in our article are just used to prove or set off our ideas within the confines of previous knowledge. We cannot always describe the sources' idea but ignore what we want to demonstrate in writing.

2.1.1.3.2　Acknowledging the sources and references. Many references and sources are searched and referred to before starting the research project and eventually publishing. We have to ensure that we select all of the references to sustain or foreshadow our academic work. Citing the references used to develop the argument based on the research findings is really necessary to a sound academic article. But every source and reference that has been used must be clearly indicated in our article, summarizing the original author's ideas. Acknowledgement of the sources and references reflects a respect to previous authors.

2.1.1.3.2.1　When should we acknowledge the source that we express in our article. It is definitely necessary to credit the source whenever any information is used from the external source, whether a snippet or entire module. Secondly, references and sources should be cited when ideas are summarized even if put in different sentence construction

2.1.1.3.2.2　How to cite the source. This is usually determined by the journal, so before making a reference citation, one should first ensure the styles that are preferred by the journal: MLA, APA and so on; for website sources the URL and the date accessed are generally sufficient; when the information is adapted, one should indicate this with the terms "adapted from" or "based upon" to help the readers understand what has been modified.

2.1.1.4　Rational use in TCM writing: The citation of the classical and ancient references is not plagiarism. The classical and ancient references are the foundation of TCM, where so many of citations are used to demonstrate the opinion of the authors. However, the sources, the name and who is the famous author of the classical reference should be described directly.

2.1.2　Self-plagiarism: Self-plagiarism is commonly described as recycling or reusing one's own specific words from previously published texts. Beyond verbatim sections of text, self-plagiarism can also refer to the publication of identical papers in two journals (sometimes called "duplicate publication"). Duplicate publication, Salami-slicing and text-recycling are common forms of the self-plagiarism. In short, self-plagiarism is any attempt to take any of your own previously published text, papers, or research results and make it appear brand new.

2.1.2.1　Duplicate publication

2.1.2.1.1　Introduction: Duplicate publication refers to an overlap in the content of a previously published work of the author. In this case, the contents of the duplicate published work might be nearly identical and have at least one common author. As one of the forms of self-plagiarism, duplicate publication is the action where one manuscript is submitted to two different journals.

There are some situations where the duplicate publication is however acceptable:

2.1.2.1.1.1　Change the language. Some journals may permit the author to republish a work in another journal using a different language. However, the new version must clearly indicate that it is a duplicate of an existing original version.

2.1.2.1.1.2　Each journal has its independent readership and do not necessarily affect others. Some authors who submit the same article to more than one journal rationalize their behavior by explaining that each journal has its own independent readership and that their duplicate paper would be of interest to each set of readers who would probably not otherwise be aware of the other publication.

2.1.2.1.2　Why should one avoid duplicate publication

2.1.2.1.2.1　Delaying the publication efficiency of papers. The publication of papers is a process that generally includes three stages: first submission review, final review and publication. Duplicate publication to the same journal or different journals leads to a repeated review of the paper, increasing the workload of the journal in regards to paper review and editing. In general, a paper can only be delivered once to any particular journal. If the author resorts to "duplicate publication", the audit process would include time to identify the repeated publication, greatly delaying the efficiency of the journal editing process.

2.1.2.1.2.2　Wasting resources. Duplicate publication results in a great waste of resources. Each journal's resources are limited. "Duplicate publication" leads to a paper occupying the journals resources, which is not conducive to maximize the use of these resources.

2.1.2.1.3　How can we avoid it. Replicating a previous article's content is the main feature of duplicate publication. So, to avoid duplicate publication, one should not copy content from previous publications other than what is essential to build one's new research upon. Such references should be clearly indicated. Here are some authoring tips that should be considered .

2.1.2.1.3.1　Do not replicate content from any of your other published papers.

2.1.2.1.3.2　Do not offer preliminary reports about unpublished papers to the media, companies, or other agencies, without the permission of the journal.

2.1.2.1.3.3　When quoting material from your previously published work, do not include more than a few sentences from the older work. Also, place the text in quotation marks and cite the source.

2.1.2.1.3.4　When using a single dataset to write more than one manuscript, ensure that: each manuscript addresses separate and important questions, the manuscripts are cross-referenced, and you inform the journal editors about this matter in a cover letter.

2.1.2.1.3.5 If you have published related papers, provide details of these papers to the journal editor at the time of submission. Include copies of these papers with the submitted manuscript. This will ensure full transparency and will help the editor make the right decision.

2.1.2.2 Salami-slicing

2.1.2.2.1 Introduction: Salami-slicing or Salami publication usually refers to submitting different manuscripts drawn from data collected from a single research study or a single data collection period. It is the action that the author divides one research into several publications without cross-reference. In this situation, each of the articles shares the same hypothesis, method and publication.

2.1.2.2.2 Why should we avoid Salami-slicing

2.1.2.2.2.1 Reduce the quality of the paper. Salami-slicing divides the same research results into multiple parts and published in different journals. Although it can increase the number of papers attributed to the author, Salami-slicing undermines the integrity of scientific research results and reduces the quality of the paper. In general, a research project revolves around a new idea, or solutions to a new problem. Researchers focus on creativity and problems in the early researches on the basis of scientific research and rigorous experimental process, and ultimately demonstrate the rationality of new ideas or provide a new way to solve the problem. Salami-slicing divides a complete scientific research process and scientific research into several parts, seriously undermining the integrity of scientific research innovation and scientific research system, leading to the analysis and demonstration of published papers too shallow, and lack of depth, and seriously reducing the quality of the paper.

2.1.2.2.2.2 Weakening the impact of research results and being not conducive to scientific research and innovation. Salami-slicing reduces the quality of the papers and brings some negative impact to their influence. Salami-slicing involves the division of research results. Although each paper may has its own dedicated discussion, the depth of its discussion is still more superficial than if a complete discussion of the paper is made. In addition, the paper divided into multiple articles, lacks or weakens the analysis from the whole study or the overall perspective in the analysis and discussion. Finally, while the readers are searching for relevant literature, there will be a big deficiency, which can result in difficulty to fully understand the theoretical results and significance of the study. Salami-slicing weakens the influence of research results.

2.1.2.2.3 How can we avoid Salami-slicing: The objective of the author when resorting to

Salami-slicing is to increase the quantity of journal publications. As to that, the measures to solve the problem should be decided by the author self. Research is a process aiming to explore the unknown world, and a publication should be the introduction to that whole research, including the data, the research method and the discussion to prove what the research has shown. As an author, one should articulate the exploration of the research in detail. One research project should ideally produce one paper that describes fully what has been found.

2.1.2.2.4　The Salami-slicing in TCM writing: Salami-slicing is one of the most common dishonesties in TCM writing. The diagnoses of the TCM differ by the cold or hot, virtual or real, Yin or Yang. So, one disease always includes several branches in TCM. In the process of the TCM research, different drugs and skills are used in some or all of the branches. This will influence many results. Some authors may sub-divide the results obtained by the different branches to increase the numbers of the articles produced by the research. So, as a TCM researcher, all of the branches should be described and demonstrated in one article to avoid Salami-slicing.

2.1.2.3　Text-recycling

2.1.2.3.1　Introduction: Text-recycling is when sections of the same text appear in more than one of the author's own publications. It is a range from an author republishing the result twice without citing, to reproduction of several sections and paragraphs of his or her own previous articles. Sometimes the author may refer to previously published material to support his new publication. But there is still no consensus about how much of the text overlap is still not assured by the editors.

There are some situations that do not belong to the text-recycling: a. Recycling from these documents [e.g., Institutional Review Board (IRB) applications, Animal Care and Use Committee applications, internal grant applications] or other forms of unpublished 'internal' documents to demonstrate more details about the background, purpose, scope and the expected results of the research. b. Reuse of the content that is not copyright in subsequent presentations/ publications targeted for wider dissemination (e.g., conference presentations, published papers). The original documents for a private entity are excepted.

2.1.2.3.2　Why should text-recycling be avoided

2.1.2.3.2.1　Confusing the readers. Readers' main focus when reading newly-published papers should be on the new idea being presented. The re-use of the text leads to the emergence and repetition of the author's old ideas in the present new paper, so that the old and new ideas may become confused. This may lead to the readers not distinguishing between the old and the new concepts.

2.1.2.3.2.2　Wasting source of publication. The principle of publishing a paper is to present new ideas from the author's new research. If the author writes more about the ideas previously published, the editorial process will spend lots of time repeating reviews. Text recycling is against the principle of writing for publication. It wastes the limited layout resources of journals.

2.1.2.3.3　How can text-recycling be avoided?

The methods to be used to avoid text cycling are still uncertain. Different journals equip different standards about the range of the overlap. The Biomed recommends editors to consider these tips when dealing with text recycling:

2.1.2.3.3.1　How much text is recycled?

2.1.2.3.3.2　Where in the article the text recycling occurs?

2.1.2.3.3.3　Whether the source of the recycled text has been acknowledged.

2.1.2.3.3.4　Whether there is a breach of copyright.

2.1.2.3.3.5　In some circumstances, text-recycling follows cultural norms at the time and place of publication.

Also, Biomed require the editors consider whether there is significant overlap with a previous publication and how significantly the degree of overlap impinges on the originality of the content for the journal's audience. While the factors discussed below should be taken into consideration when deciding on the significance of the overlap, editors need to decide whether the author has re-used text legitimately or has misrepresented previously presented ideas or data as new. According to the standards of the Biomed, the quantity of the recycled text should be limited to requirements set by Biomed for its potential authors.

Besides the Biomed, other journals have their own standard to identify and deal with the text recycling. So, there is no common standard or tips that adapted to every journal in this world. But some contents are similar: the quantity of the overlap and the copyrights of the overlap. Still, we ought to decide and identify the text recycling by the journal we will publish when writing medical papers.

2.2　Fabrication or falsification

2.2.1　Introduction: Berkeley city college defines " fabrication " as " the falsification of data, information, or citations in any formal academic exercise." Proper citation of references is generally addressed by the assigned or adopted writing-style manual. Occasionally, however, papers are submitted with false references. Fabrication or falsification is the action of articulating the information of the research separating from the truth of the research. Trumping up the survey data, and figures, and concocting the references' opinion are the most common behaviors in the fabrication or falsification.

2.2.2 Why should fabrication be avoided

2.2.2.1 Self-credibility is seriously damaged. Academic "fraud" seriously affected the author's "credibility". Unlike plagiarism, the negative effects of the misconduct are greater and more severe. In medical research, "fabrication" may cause serious harm to human health, so many institutions take "fabrication" seriously and punishment is more stringent.

2.2.2.2 Being not conducive to the construction of disciplines and innovation. The purpose of scientific research is to enhance the discipline of innovation and development. New scientific research design, practice and analysis of the argument must be related to other authors of the relevant research as an important basis for argument. The academic fabrication in medical research would provide a wrong guidance for any follow-up study, which leads to the deviation of the development direction of the related fields of the subject and hinders the correct development of the discipline.

2.2.2.3 Endangering public health. Medical scientific research provides some correct guidance for the health of the public. The "fabrication" misconduct in medical research not only affects the innovation and development of the discipline, but also can cause great harm to public health. The main purpose of medical research is to explore new concepts in etiology, pathogenesis and treatment of the disease through the scientific experimental design. By the detailed description of the medical science research and the logical demonstration analysis of the feasibility of the purpose of the study, medical papers provide the direction about health. Medical staff, in the diagnosis and treatment of the disease, often considers the guidance in journals as an important reference to understand a disease and identify the latest and most effective treatment to improve the cure rate of patients with the disease. Trumping up the results of the study, the methods of the study, the sample size, and the interventions would cause serious misleading to the medical treatment of the clinician and some serious harm to the health of the public.

2.2.3 How can falsification be avoided? Minimize the opportunity for an allegation of academic dishonesty for using false references by incorporating the following into your preparation:

2.2.3.1　Allow sufficient time to thoroughly research and gather all information necessary for proper citation and reference format.

2.2.3.2　Learn what the prescribed writing style requires for references and use it.

2.2.3.3　Double check the completed document with your research notes for accuracy.

3. Citation

Citation is signing and specifying the source in the writing process, which can help the readers to return to the original literature again according to the information the paper provided. Generally, citing a reference includes author's information, thesis title, journal name, publication date and page number where the paper is located. Citation is an important way to avoid "plagiarism".

3.1　Necessity of citation

3.1.1　To facilitate the reader to be able to trace the source of the arguments and determine whether the original literature argument is correct. It is an important function of citation. Readers in the process of reading papers, sometimes need to return to the original papers to search for the information and materials they need. Reference citation can help readers to identify the original literature to facilitate the continuation of the relevant research materials collection. In addition, the reader in the process of reading may need to return to the original data to determine whether the original data is reasonable or whether the arguments are correct. The citation index can help the reader review the original data and determine whether the paper is accurate and whether the original data arguments are correct.

3.1.2　To support the views of the paper. The demonstration of the paper's idea needs some correct references to support the literature. Citation can clearly present the source and evidence cited in the process of argumentation. In addition, citation can clearly distinguish between the literature view and the author's own point of view, which is more conducive to help the author to achieve creativity and results of the argument.

3.2　When to cite　Whenever we borrow the words or the ideas from others, we ought to cite the references. The citation must be annotated in the follow situations:

3.2.1　Quoting the other's words or sentences.

3.2.2　Paraphrasing other's idea or sentences.

3.2.3 Using the ideas that have been articulated.

3.2.4 Making specific reference to the research method of another.

3.2.5 Some previous concept that makes a great difference to the new idea being proposed.

3.3 How to cite without misconduct The literature reference is the only way to solve "plagiarism". In the paper cited in the literature, the author not only pays attention to the literature cited with the format requirements, but also tries to avoid "plagiarism" through reasonable means. The following entries are effective means of avoiding "plagiarism".

3.3.1 Paraphrasing the sources and avoiding direct copying. In the literature citation, articulating the original data in our voice is a commonly used means to reduce the repetition rate. Paraphrasing methods include: a. Change the sentence structure. b. Synonyms replace the words that are not generically used. c. Active and passive tones exchange. d. Expression exchange. e. Change part of the topic.

3.3.2 Quote directly: directly quote the words or sentences after the quotation marks, and determine the source of the literature.

4. Suggesting Reading After Class

So many academic integrity and misconduct have been focused by the universities and colleges all over the world. Some journals also build their own standards. In the USA, the Office of Research Integrity of the Department of Human health Service (DHHS) has promulgated the *Duplicate Publication*. This regulation of the DHHS describes so many details about the misconduct and integrity.

Duplicate Publication (DHHS): It will help you identify the dishonesty in medical writing for publication comprehensively.

5. Homework

Homework 1 Compare the styles of the plagiarism and identify the difference with each other.

Homework 2 Search 3 journals' standard about the text recycling and write an essay about your opinion on how to avoid the text recycling.

References

[1] University of Pennsylvania. Avoiding Plagiarism: When in Doubt, Cite [EB/OL]. [2017 - 04 - 13]. http://www.upenn.edu/academicintegrity/ai_citingsources.html.

[2] DHHS. Duplicate Publication [EB/OL]. [2017 - 04 - 07]. http://ori.hhs.gov/plagiarism-14.

[3] Editage Insight. Duplicate publications and simultaneous submissions [EB/OL]. [2017 - 04 - 14]. http://www.editage.com/insights/duplicate-publications-and-simultaneous-submissions.

[4] COPE. Texting Recycling [EB/OL]. [2017 - 04 - 18]. https://publicationethics.org/files/Web_A29298_COPE_Text_Recycling.

[5] Berkerly City College. What is academic dishonesty? [EB/OL]. [2017 - 04 - 15]. http://www.berkeleycitycollege.edu/wp/de/what-is-academic-dishonesty.

[6] UTDALLAS. Academic Dishonesty [EB/OL]. [2017 - 04 - 14]. http://www.utdallas.edu/conduct/dishonesty.

第三章 中医辨证分析在病案中的应用

中医临床诊治疾病,既辨病又辨证,主要是将重点放在"证"的区别上,通过辨证而进一步认识疾病,从而提出治疗方案。因此在病案书写中需要通过条理清晰的辨证分析得到疾病的病名和证型。分析、综合、判断,是辨证诊断过程中基本的思维形式,也是病案中辨证分析书写的要点。

目前中医病案中,在主诉、病史采集描述后,中医诊断中的病名基本确定后,中医证型的确定需要辨证分析,因此辨证分析是病案中重要且关键的一部分。

中医临床"辨证论治"过程示意图如图3-1。

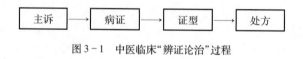

图3-1 中医临床"辨证论治"过程

一、病案中辨证分析的要点

(1)辨清病因、病位、病机。

(2)提出类证鉴别的思路与依据。

(3)评估病情的发展、预后。

二、病案中辨证的概念及分析过程

1. 病与证的概念

(1)病:是对疾病整个过程规律所作的概括。一个病可有几个证的演变过程。比如肾病,有不同的证候,如肾气虚、肾阴虚、肾阳虚。

(2)证:在确认"病"的基础上再进行"证"的分析,是对疾病发展过程中某一阶段病理概括。

（3）辨证：是中医治疗的基础,中医医生需要诊断出"病"和"证"。把四诊的记述加以综合,在阴阳、五行、脏腑、经络理论基础上,找出疾病的病因病机,从而阐述疾病的病理本质。

2. 如何辨证 辨主要症状：围绕对主症的辨别,明确疾病的病因、病机、病位。

（1）需要了解主要症状与证候的联系,有些症状具有直接确定证候的作用。

如主症为"咳嗽的患者",伴有恶寒发热、脉浮——表证;伴重、浊、腻、渴不欲饮——湿;若同时伴形体肥胖——痰湿;若伴苔黄腻,脉濡数或滑数——湿热或痰热。

（2）部分症状的辨证：如虚证的诊断——神疲、体倦、乏力、脉虚为气虚。

心气虚＝气虚+心悸、怔忡。

肺气虚＝气虚+咳嗽、喘息。

脾气虚＝气虚+食少、腹胀、便溏。

肾气虚＝气虚+腰膝酸软。

三、辨证分析的步骤

1. 问病史 一般疾病,都有感受冷热、饮食不节、情志受伤等病史,应根据情况首先询问,若经询问确实无明显诱因发病,亦应描述。

2. 审证求因 根据症状特点、性质等探求其发生的原因。

3. 确定病位 就是辨别病变的主要部位。病位是指病变所在的部位,一般用表里、脏腑等表示。外感病多用表里、脏腑、卫气营血、三焦等表示,杂病多用脏腑、气血阴阳等表示。

4. 审察病机 病因侵及一定的部位,则有一定的病机,根据脉征的变化可审察明确病机的变化。

5. 分清病性 在明确病机的同时,要知病情之所属。主要根据八纲辨证,辨别疾病的寒热虚实等病性。如口渴喜冷饮,尿赤便结,脉数为热;口淡不渴或喜热饮,尿清便溏,脉迟为寒。

6. 详析病势 病势即病机转变发展的趋势。判断病势,主要根据脉征的变化进行分析。如阳证脉势减缓,表示邪气渐退,为病将愈。

7. 确定证名 证候的命名,一般以病因、病位、病机三者综合最佳,如脾虚湿滞、肺热痰壅等。由于证候诊断与疾病诊断常同时进行,因此证型名和病名也常同时确定。第一诊断中医病名与主诉须对应。

四、辨证的综合运用

1. 八纲辨证与脏腑辨证方法 八纲是辨证的总纲,用八纲来分析和归纳。但这不能反映疾病的本质,还须结合脏腑辨证来分析其本质。

2. 外感病与内伤病的辨证

(1)外感病的辨证方法有六经辨证、卫气营血辨证、三焦辨证等。

(2)杂病的辨证方法有脏腑辨证、气血津液辨证、经络辨证等。

五、辨病、类证鉴别与类病鉴别

1. 疾病诊断的定名 辨病是指疾病诊断,也称病名诊断。

2. 疾病诊断的依据

(1)辨病的依据就是所给病案患者现病史中的第一个症状或主要症状。如:咳嗽则辨病是咳嗽,心悸心慌则是心悸,心前区憋闷疼痛则为胸痹心痛。

(2)有些复杂的疾病的辨病就要靠掌握该病的临床特点。如:肺痨则是咳嗽、咳痰、咯血、低热、盗汗。肺炎喘嗽:热、咳、痰、喘、煽五症具备。

3. 疾病的鉴别诊断 某些疾病容易混淆,应注意鉴别。如癫、狂、痫三种虽同是神志异常的疾病,但各有其症状特点。癫病者以沉默痴呆、语无伦次、静而多喜为特征;狂病者以躁妄打骂、喧扰不宁、动而多怒为特征;痫病者以猝然昏倒、不省人事、四肢抽搐、口吐涎沫、口中作如猪、羊叫声为特征。

六、辨病与辨证的关系

证和病两者有密切的关系。如感冒病,其证有风寒证和风热证的不同,须用不同的治法;再如头痛与眩晕虽属两病但均可出现血虚证候。因此,既要辨证,又要辨病。

"病"是从辨证而得的,一种病有一种病的变化规律,这个"病"的规律,又反过来指导辨证。辨证—辨病—辨证,是一个诊断疾病不断深化的过程。

因此,我们不能只以辨证为满足,必须既辨证,又辨病,由辨病再进一步辨证,两者不可偏废。在病案书写中需要通过条理清晰的辨证分析从而得到疾病的病名和证型,即中医辨证分析在病案中的应用。

七、外感病及内伤病辨证思路例举

(一)外感病:"咳嗽"

(1)明确诊断为"咳嗽病",辨清"外感"或"内伤",见表3-1。

表 3-1 外感咳嗽与内伤咳嗽辨证要点

辨证要点	外 感 咳 嗽	内 伤 咳 嗽
病程	短	长
起病方式	快	慢
表证	有	无
诱因	外感风寒、风热、风燥	饮食、情志、素有肺系疾病

（2）外感咳嗽辨"风寒""风热""风燥"，见图 3-2。

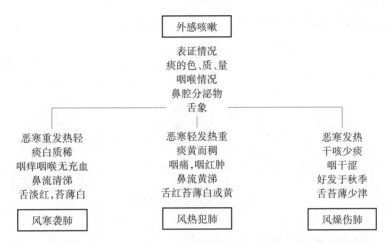

图 3-2 外感咳嗽辨证要点

（3）内伤咳嗽辨清脏腑，见图 3-3。

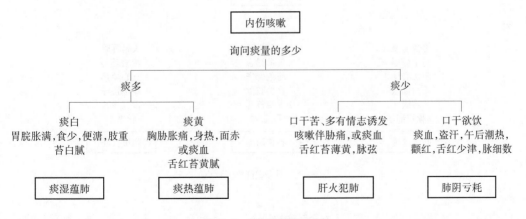

图 3-3 内伤咳嗽辨证要点

（二）内伤病："不寐"

（1）明确诊断为"不寐"病。辨别"虚证"与"实证"，见表 3-2。

表3-2 实证不寐与虚证不寐辨证要点

辨证要点	不 寐 实 证	不 寐 虚 证
病程	短	长
症状和体征	体质壮实,伴心烦易怒,口苦咽干,便秘溲赤	体质瘦弱,伴面色少华,神疲懒言,心悸健忘
脉象	脉弦滑,数而有力	脉细软弱,数而无力

（2）脏腑辨证

1）不寐实证辨证要点,见图3-4。

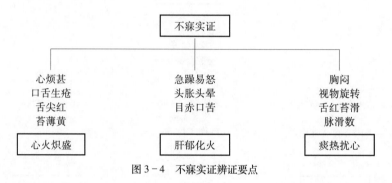

图3-4 不寐实证辨证要点

2）不寐虚证辨证要点,见图3-5。

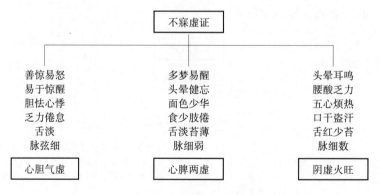

图3-5 不寐虚证辨证要点

八、病例分析

李某,男,46岁,职员。2018年1月7日冬季就诊。

患者于3日前因天气变化受凉后出现恶寒发热,无汗,头痛,肢节酸疼,鼻塞声重,鼻痒喷嚏,时流清涕,咽痒,咽痛,咳嗽,痰吐稀薄色白,渴喜热饮,遂来就诊。舌苔薄白而润,脉浮紧。

（1）根据上述摘要,完成辨证分析。

（2）中医类证鉴别,请与时行感冒鉴别。

病案辨证分析部分可参考如下。

1）中医疾病诊断:感冒(风寒束表证)。

2）中医辨病辨证依据(含病因病机分析):① 辨病依据:患者因气候变凉诱发,出现恶寒发热,无汗,鼻塞,流涕,喷嚏,咽痒,咽痛,中医辨病为感冒。② 辨证依据:无汗,头痛,肢节酸疼,鼻塞声重,鼻痒喷嚏,时流清涕,咽痒,痰吐稀薄色白,渴喜热饮,舌苔薄白而润,脉浮紧为风寒束表证。

3）病因病机分析:外出受凉,感受寒邪,风寒外束,卫阳被郁,腠理闭塞,肺气不宣。病位在卫表肺系,病性属表属实。

4）中医类证鉴别:本病可与时行感冒鉴别。时行感冒病情较重,发病急,全身症状显著,具有广泛的传染性、流行性。而普通感冒病情较轻,全身症状不重,少有传变,无明显流行特点。因此该患者诊断为"感冒",当属"风寒束表"。

参考文献

[1] 陈湘君.中医内科常见病证辨证思路与方法[M].北京:人民卫生出版社,2003.

Chapter Three

TCM Clinical Thinking and Medical Record Writing

The process of TCM diagnosis is the combination of disease identification and syndrome identification with more emphasis being placed on syndrome identification which is used for further stratification of identifying disease and guiding treatment. So, in medical record writing, we need to document a clear syndrome identification analysis to identify the disease and TCM syndrome. Therefore, analysis, synthesis, and judgment are the basic thought processes of syndrome identification and the main point in medical records as well.

In TCM medical records, when the chief complaint and medical history are already provided and disease name is confirmed, we need syndrome identification analysis to confirm TCM pattern. Therefore, syndrome identification analysis is the important and key part in medical record.

The diagram of syndrome identification and treatment is as follows (Figure 3 − 1):

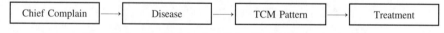

Figure 3 − 1 The diagram of syndrome identification and treatment

1. The Main Points of Syndrome Identification Analysis in Medical Records

1.1 Identify the cause, location, and pathogenesis.

1.2 Propose the thought and basis of differential diagnosis.

1.3 Assess the disease progression and prognosis.

2. Syndrome Identification Concept and Analysis Process in Medical Records

2.1 The concept of disease and syndrome

2.1.1 Disease refers to the entire course of pathological changes whereas the name of a syndrome reflects the pathology of a disease at a certain stage. For example, in a disease arising from a kidney disorder, the syndrome may involve Yang-deficiency, Yin-deficiency or Qi-deficiency, etc.

2.1.2　Syndrome thus refers to a complex pattern of signs and symptoms that manifest at a given stage of the disease.

2.1.3　Syndrome identification is the premise and foundation of TCM treatment. A TCM practitioner will diagnose both the disease and the syndrome. Syndrome identification is the comprehensive analysis of clinical information gained by the four-main diagnostic TCM procedures and is based on Yin and Yang, five elements, the viscera and the meridian theory to identify the causes and pathogenesis of the disease and describe the disease pathological nature.

2.2　How to identify the syndrome　Identify the main symptoms: the cause of disease, pathogenesis and location.

Example 1: Understand the relationship between the main symptoms and TCM pattern. Some symptoms can confirm TCM pattern directly. Such as the main symptom is "cough" — if accompanied by aversion to cold and fever, and floating pulse implies exterior syndrome; if accompanied by heaviness, turbidity, greasy, and thirst without desire for drink implies wet syndrome; if accompanied by physical obesity implies phlegm dampness; if accompanied by yellow tongue coating and slippery or rapid pulse implies dampness heat or phlegm heat.

Example 2: Localized symptoms syndrome identification such as the diagnosis of deficiency syndrome — mental and physical lassitude, fatigue, pulse deficiency implies Qi deficiency. However,

Heart Qi deficiency = Qi deficiency + palpitations

Lung Qi deficiency = Qi deficiency + cough, shortness of breath

Spleen Qi deficiency = Qi deficiency + poor appetite, abdomen distention, loose stools

Kidney Qi deficiency = Qi deficiency + soreness and weakness of waist and knees.

3. The Steps of Syndrome Identification Analysis

3.1　Medical history taking　Generally, diseases have some common medical history like getting cold, unhealthy diet and emotional injuries, which should be enquired about based on different situations. If there is no obvious causation of the disease in medical history, this should also be described in medical record.

3.2　Differentiating symptoms and sign to identify cause　To find out the causes of disease onset according to the characteristics and nature of the symptoms.

3.3　Confirming the location of disease　To identify the main location of the disease, which refers to the location of the disease described by internal and external theory or viscera theory. Exogenous diseases often use the internal and external, the viscera, Wei-Qi-Yin-blood, or the Sanjiao theory to be described. The endogenous diseases are often described by viscera, Qi and blood, and Yin and Yang.

3.4　Examine pathogenesis　If a cause invades a certain part, this would be associated with a defined pathogenesis, and the progression can be examined according to the change of the pulse sign.

3.5　Identify the nature of the disease　confirm the pathogenesis and the location of disease. It is mainly based on eight diagnostic principle to distinguish the disease from cold and heat, and excess and deficiency. For example, thirst with the desire of cold drink, reddish coloured urine and constipation, and a rapid pulse imply heat syndrome; bland taste in the mouth without the desire to drink or desiring hot drink, clear urine and loose stool, and a slow pulse imply cold syndrome.

3.6　Detailed analysis of the disease　the trend and progression of the disease reflect the pathogenesis, which is mainly based on the changes of symptoms and pulse sign. If the pulse slows down in Yang syndrome, it means that the evil Qi is gradually receding, and the disease will be cured.

3.7　Confirming TCM pattern name　The naming of the syndrome is generally based on the cause, the location of disease, and the pathogenesis, such as spleen deficiency with dampness, and lung heat due to phlegm. Syndrome name and disease name are often confirmed together. The first TCM diagnosis must correspond to chief complain.

4. The Comprehensive Application of Syndrome Identification

4.1　The Eight principle syndrome identification and viscera syndrome identification　The eight principle is the general outline of syndrome identification and is used to analyze and summarize disease. However, this classification does not reflect the nature of the disease. Eight principle syndrome identification must be used with combination of viscera syndrome identification.

4.2 Syndrome identification of exogenous diseases and endogenous diseases

4.2.1 The syndrome identification of exogenous diseases includes six-meridians, Wei-Qi-Yin-xue, and Sanjiao syndrome identification.

4.2.2 The syndrome identification of endogenous diseases includes viscera, Qi-blood-liquid-fluid, and meridians syndrome identification.

5. Identification of Diseases, Syndrome Identification and Differential Diagnosis

5.1 Confirm the disease name the disease diagnosis refers to diagnosing disease, also called the diagnosis of the disease name.

5.2 The basis for disease diagnosis

5.2.1 Diagnosing the disease is based on the chief complain or the main symptom in patients' medical history. Thus if the symptom is cough so the disease diagnosis is cough; if the presenting symptom is palpitations so the disease diagnosis is palpitations; and if the symptom is heart pain in the anterior area so the disease diagnosis is chest pain.

5.2.2 Diagnosing some complicated diseases depends on the clinical characteristics of the disease. For example, lung consumption manifests as dry cough, hemoptysis, low fever, and night sweats. Pneumonia manifests as fever, cough, phlegm, panting, and nasal flaring.

5.3 Differential diagnosis Some diseases share similar symptoms and signs which should be differentiated. For example, psychosis, mania, and epilepsy belong to spiritual abnormal diseases, but each one has its own features. Psychosis is characterized by silent dementia, incoherent speech, and more joyful with silence. Mania is characterized by manic agitation with excessive movement and anger. Epilepsy is characterized by faint, unconsciousness, twitching in the extremities, vomiting in the mouth, and the sound like pigs and sheep in the mouth.

6. The Relationship Between Disease Identification and Syndrome Identification

There is a close relationship between the syndrome and the disease. For example, common cold disease involves wind-cold syndrome and wind-heat syndrome which deserve different treatments. Headache and dizziness are two different diseases, but they can be having the same TCM pattern — blood deficiency syndrome. Therefore, it is necessary to combine disease identification with syndrome identification.

The "disease" is obtained from syndrome identification. A disease has its own rule of change which in turn guides syndrome identification. Syndrome identification — identifying disease — symptom identification is a process of diagnosing diseases.

Therefore, we must combine syndrome identification with diseases identification and start from disease identification to guide syndrome identification further. In writing medical records, it is necessary to obtain the disease name and syndrome pattern through well-organized analysis, which is the application of TCM syndrome identification analysis in medical records.

7. Exogenous Disease and Endogenous Disease Syndrome Identification

7.1 Exogenous disease: cough

7.1.1 Confirming diagnosis: "cough disease" (Table 3 - 1).

Table 3 - 1 Differentia "exogenous cough" or "endogenous cough"

Diagnostic points	Exogenous cough	Endogenous cough
Duration	Short	Long
Onset	Sudden	Chronic
Exterior signs	Present	Absent
Causes	External wind-cold, wind-heat, wind-dryness	Diet、emotions、chronic lung diseases

7.1.2 Differentiate wind-cold, wind-heat, wind-dry (Figure 3 - 2).

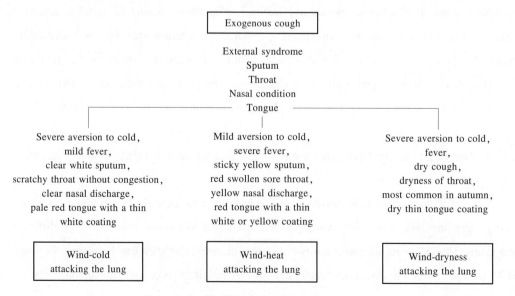

Figure 3 - 2 The dialectical points of exogenous cough

7.1.3 Differentiate endogenous cough (Figure 3 − 3).

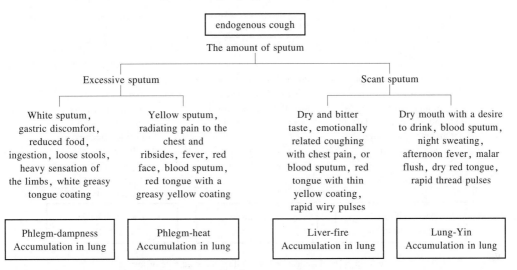

Figure 3 − 3 The dialectical points of endogenous cough

7.2 Endogenous disease: insomnia

7.2.1 Confirming diagnosis: insomnia (Table 3 − 2)

Table 3 − 2 Differentiate syndrome from "excess syndrome" or "deficiency syndrome"

Diagnostic points	Excess	Deficiency
Duration	Short	Long
Constitution sign and symptom	Excess constitution with heart vexation, irascibility, bitter taste in the mouth, dry throat, constipation, reddish urine	Weak constitution with lusterless complexion, fatigue, reticence, palpitations
Pulse	Wiry, slippery, forceful and rapid	Thin, rapid and weak

7.2.2 Viscera syndrome identification

7.2.2.1 Excess syndrome (Figure 3 − 4).

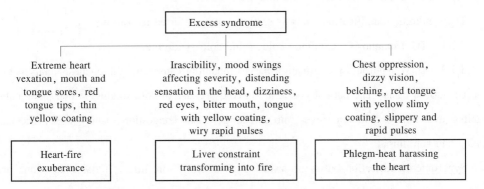

Figure 3 − 4 The dilectical points of excess syndrome of insomnia

7.2.2.2   Deficiency syndrome (Figure 3 - 5).

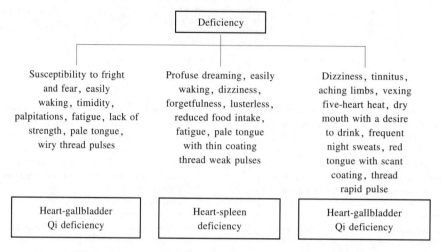

Figure 3 - 5   The dilectical points of dificiency syndrome of insomnia

8. Clinical Case

Li, male, 46 years old, staff member. January 07, 2018 winter visit.

The patient developed cold and fever after experiencing weather changes 3 days ago. His reported symptomatology included no sweating, headache, sore limbs, nasal congestion, nasal itching, sneezing, itchy and sore throat, cough, vomiting thin white sputum, and a desire for warm drinks. On examination, the tongue is white thin and moist, and the pulse is tight and floating.

8.1   Complete the syndrome identification analysis according to the case

8.2   Differential diagnosis with influenza

The syndrome identification analysis section can be referred as follow:

8.2.1   TCM diagnosis   Common cold, wind-cold syndrome.

8.2.2   TCM syndrome identification basis (including cause and pathogenesis analysis):

Diagnostic basis: The patient got common cold because of cold weather which made patient manifest aversion to cold and fever, no sweating, nasal congestion, runny nose, sneezing, itching and sore throat.

Syndrome identification basis: no sweating, headache, sore limbs, nasal congestion, nasal itching, sneezing, itchy throat, thin white sputum, thirsty with desiring drink, thin white and moist tongue coating, and floating tight pulse imply wind-cold syndrome.

8.2.3 Analysis of cause and pathogenesis The patient who got cold outside was attacked by evil cold. The cold wind made the Wei-yang depressed and lung-qi blocked. The location of the disease is in the exterior so the nature of the disease is exterior excess syndrome.

8.2.4 Differential diagnosis of TCM syndromes This disease can be compared with influenza. Influenza is relatively severe, acute and the systemic symptoms are relatively more significant and it has a wide range of contagious and epidemic characteristics. The common cold is mild, the systemic symptoms are not that heavy and there are less changeable than influenza and there is no obvious epidemic characteristics. Therefore, the patient is diagnosed as a "common cold with cold-wind syndrome".

References

[1] Chen XJ. Thoughts and methods of syndrome differentiation of common diseases and syndromes in internal medicine of traditional Chinese medicine [M]. Beijing: People's Health Publishing House, 2003.

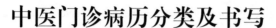

第四章 中医门诊病历分类及书写

中医门诊病历可能是我们最早接触的病历种类。回顾既往,主要有以下三种形式:实录式医案、追忆式医案以及病历式医案。

一、概述

1. **实录式医案** 流行于清代的实录式医案为医家门诊或出诊时当场留下的文字资料,也被我们称之为"案"。前为议论,称为案语,后为药物,一般写在处方笺上。

2. **追忆式医案** 追忆式医案,又称之为"医话性医案"。为医者诊后追忆诊疗的过程、效果、副作用,然后笔之于书的文字资料。

3. **病历式医案** 病历是用来描述一个患者的医疗史和护理在特定的医疗保健提供者的管辖范围内的一个系统文件。医疗记录包括各种类型的"记录",随着时间的推移,由医疗保健专业人士记录观察、给药和治疗、药品管理和治疗的规则、测试结果等。

近代一些中医仿照西医病历的格式,分项记述患者一般情况、症状、病理、诊断、疗法、处方、效果等,分类清楚,记载较为全面。这种医案,称之为病历式医案。

4. **实录式医案、追忆式医案、病历式医案三者关系** 见图 4-1。

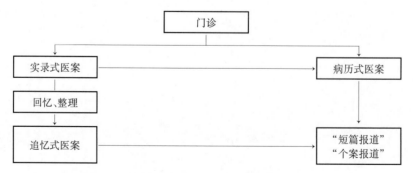

图 4-1 实录式医案、追忆式医案、病历式医案三者关系

二、实录式医案

1. 实录式医案特点 病情记录比较真实,药物、剂量、炮制等项目亦能详细记录,能忠实反映医家诊疗的原貌。

2. 著名实录式医案 《临证指南医案》《未刻本叶氏医案》《柳选四家医案》《丁甘仁医案》和《清代名医医案精华》等均是这类格式。

3. 实录式医案的种类

(1) 先述症状,后分析病因病机,然后下诊断、出治法者。如《丁甘仁医案》王妪案:

症状:寒热,呕恶,饮食不进,腹痛痢下,日夜五六十次,赤白相杂,里急后重,舌苔腻布,脉象浮紧而数。

病因病机:感受时气之邪,袭于表分,湿热夹滞,互阻肠胃。

诊断:噤口痢之重症。

治疗原则:先宜解表导滞。

方药:荆芥5克,防风3克,豆豉9克,薄荷3克,半夏6克,枳实5克,桔梗3克,赤芍5克,神曲9克,焦楂9克,生姜2片,红茶3克,藿香梗5克,苏梗5克,玉枢丹。

(2) 先述病机,后述症状者。如《柳选四家医案·尤在泾医案》案:

病机:病从少阳,郁入厥阴,复从厥阴,逆攻阳明。

症状:寒热往来,色青,巅顶及少腹痛,此其峰也。

治则:泄厥阴之实,顾阳明之虚,此其治也。

处方:左金丸合逍遥散。

人参,柴胡,川连,陈皮,半夏,黄芩,吴萸,茯苓,甘草。

(3) 重在分析病状之所以然,抓住主因,从而得出结论。如《柳选四家医案·尤在泾医案》案:

胁疼遇春即发,过之即止,此肝病也。春三月肝木司令,肝阳方张,而阴不能从,则其气有不达之处,故痛;夏秋冬肝气就衰,与阴适协,故不痛也。

处方:阿胶,白芍,茯苓,丹皮,茜草,甘草,鲍鱼汤代水。

(4) 症状、病因、病机、诊断、治法等结合在一起,夹叙夹论者。

如《临证指南医案》蔡妪案:

凡论病,先论体质、形色、脉象,以病乃外加于身也。夫肌肉柔白属气虚,外似丰溢,里真大怯。盖阳虚之体,为多湿多痰。

人参,半夏,生术,枳实,茯苓,生姜。

三、追忆式医案

1. 追忆式医案特点　诊疗过程及疗效记载比较清楚。有的医案有医家的辨证用药体会，文字较为生动，易读好懂。这种医案多是医家平时所遇的比较有学术价值或体会较深的病例，他们总结整理的，故常常作为作者论著的佐证或阐述作者的某一个学术观点。这类医案除单独出版外，更多地散见于医论医著中。

2. 追忆式医案的种类

（1）简略记叙疾病治疗的过程，较少议论，多为治验。宋、金、元、明的医著中多见此类医案。如《普济本事方》许叔微医案：

乡里有姓京者，以鬻绳为业，子年三十。初得病身微汗，脉弱恶风，医以麻黄药与之，汗遂不止，发热，必多惊悸，夜不得眠，谵语不识人，筋惕肉瞤，振振动摇。医者又进惊风药，予曰：此强汗之过也。仲景云：脉微弱汗出恶风者，不可服大青龙汤，服之则筋惕肉瞤，此为逆也。唯真武汤可救，进此三服，佐以清心丸，竹叶汤送下，数日愈。

（2）详细记述医者辨证论治的过程和经验体会。如《治验回忆录》案：

钟大满，腹痛有年，理中、四逆辈皆已服之，间或可止。但病发不常，或一月数发，或两月一发，每痛多为饮食寒冷之所诱致。自常以胡椒末用姜汤冲服，痛得暂解。一日，彼晤余戚家，谈其痼疾之异，乞为诊之。脉沉而弦紧，舌白润无苔。按其腹有微痛，痛时牵及腰胁，大便间日一次，少而不畅，小便如常。吾曰：君病属阴寒积聚，非温不能已其寒，非下不能荡其积，是宜温下并行。而前服理中辈无功者，仅祛寒而不逐积耳！依吾法两剂可愈。彼曰：吾固知先生善治异疾，倘得愈，感且不忘。即书于大黄附子汤：大黄，乌附，细辛。

四、病历式医案

1. 病历式医案历史　自近代著名医家张锡纯所著的《医学衷中参西录》出现之后，医案的形式变得相对固定，形成了当今病历式医案的雏形。

2. 病历式医案的框架

（1）时间日期。

（2）身份识别信息：患者姓名、年龄、职业等。

（3）主诉。

（4）现病史。

（5）十问歌（源于张景岳，由陈修园修改）。

一问寒热二问汗,三问头身四问便,

五问饮食六问胸,七聋八渴俱当辨,

九问旧病十问因,再兼服药参机变,

妇人尤必问经期,迟速闭崩皆可见,

再添片语告儿科,天花麻疹全占验。

（6）简要系统回顾。

（7）舌脉：舌,舌体大小、颜色、舌苔、舌体运动。脉：寸—关—尺（双侧）。

（8）诊断：中医诊断,病名（证型）。西医诊断。

（9）治疗原则。

（10）处方。

（11）医生签名。

3. 问病史

（1）何为病史：病史是医生通过询问患者或可以给出患者适当信息的人（认识该患者）特定的问题,目的是获得有用的信息,以给出诊断和提供医疗服务。

（2）如何写主诉：主诉是患者此次就诊最明显的症状及时间。主诉不超过20字,应该用患者的语言表述,而非专业术语。比如用"胸痛"而非"绞痛"。

当医生询问患者症状时,患者通常用自己的语言去表述痛苦及不适,医生需要通过他们的表述来提炼信息。

例如：我是好几个月前就不舒服了。一开始,我只是觉得有点不舒服,有点累。但是最近我感觉一天下来已经筋疲力尽了。我现在吃东西不多,但我从去年起重了9千克。我的行动不方便,而且我开始脱发。

主诉：乏力逐渐加重3个月,伴脱发。

其他表达主诉的方式见表4-1：

表4-1 表达主诉方式对比

建 议	不 建 议
胸痛2小时	患者胸部疼痛2小时
波动/持续高热2日	39摄氏度两日
恶心呕吐3日	患者一开始觉得自己恶心,然后每日都吐大量胃内容物大概3日
头痛1个月	患者说她头痛1个月

（3）如何收集现病史：现病史是对患者主诉更为详细的描述,是病史中最为重要的组成部分。通常医生会收集如下信息：诱因、部位、性质、持续时间、程度、发作频率、发作时

间、加重缓解因素、伴随症状等。此外还包括之前的就诊经历,如何时何地于何处就诊、诊断、实验室检查、治疗、治疗效果等。

以疼痛举例(表4－2):

表4－2　疼痛常用问题

特　征	常　用　问　题
主要部位	痛在哪里
放射痛	有没有觉得痛放射到其他地方
性质	能否描述一下痛?(灼痛、绞痛、像咬一样地痛、抓痛、锐痛、刺痛、跳痛)
诱因	痛有什么原因吗
发作时间	痛一次大概多久
频率	多久痛一次
加重因素	有什么会加重疼痛
缓解因素	有什么办法让痛好些吗
伴随症状	痛的时候有没有其他地方觉得不舒服的?有没有和疼痛相关的其他问题
持续时间	一般疼痛持续多久
严重程度	有多严重

医生需要关注到一些与疾病相关的问题,如:

1)先天因素:早产、产伤、先天畸形、遗传性疾病。

2)情志刺激:环境改变、缺少关心及陪伴、情绪问题。

3)不期因素:意外伤害、高处坠落、不慎落水、烧伤、异物吸入。

4)其他因素:环境(雾霾、吸烟、装修)、食物(激素)。

又如:着凉后流清涕,食不洁食物后腹痛及泄泻,父亲吸烟后孩子的咳嗽及哮喘。

(4)如何书写既往史、过敏史及个人史:既往史包括湿疹、哮喘、营养不良、佝偻病等病史。医生还需要写下有关哮喘、过敏性疾病、代谢性疾病和过敏(包括药物和食物)的家族史。

(5)如何写舌诊:舌头是整个身体的缩影,反映了体内的不足及过剩。舌头的形状、颜色、外皮、质地可以表明消化问题和身体不平衡。

检查标准:一个正常健康的舌头是粉红色的,薄白苔,并且舌头大小与嘴相称。新生儿舌头是红色的,没有舌苔。吃东西和吃药会影响舌诊,所以需要漱口。医生要在自然光线下观测舌头。舌头的不同部位对应着不同的器官(图4－2、图4－3)。

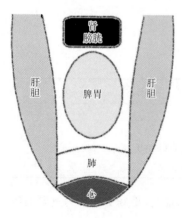

图4－2　舌头不同部位对应的器官

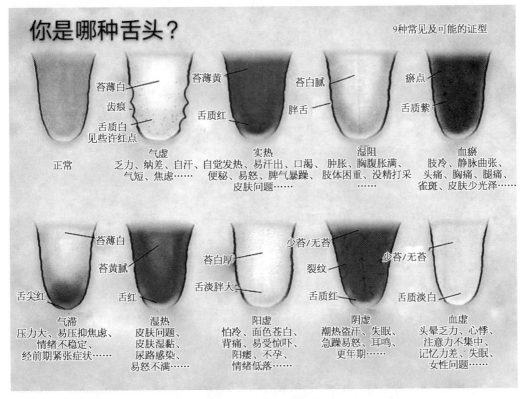

图 4 - 3 舌头的不同形态

1）舌：① 舌体胖大：阳虚。② 舌紫暗：血瘀。③ 舌淡：气血亏虚。④ 猩红舌：营血炽热。

2）舌苔：① 黄腻：湿热。② 剥苔：阴虚。

五、如何写处方

（1）中药（包括中药名、剂量及汤剂服用方法）：君，即在处方中对处方的主症或主病起主要治疗作用的药物。臣，是辅助君药加强治疗主病和主症的药物。佐，治疗主病和主症的药物。用以消除或减缓君药、臣药的毒性或烈性的药物。使，引方中诸药直达病所的药物，调和诸药。

（2）其他：针灸、艾灸、火罐、传统中医药熏蒸、导引（八段锦、五禽戏）（图 4 - 4）。

包括治疗的频率，何时实施治疗（子午流注学说）。

（3）格式

1）中药：中药一____克，中药二____克，中药三____克，中药四____克，中药五____克，

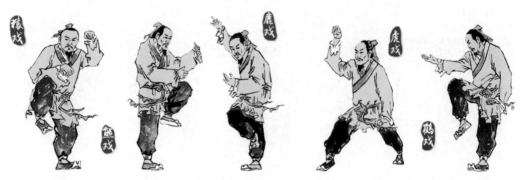

图4-4　五禽戏

中药六＿＿＿克,中药七＿＿＿克,中药八＿＿＿克,……＿＿＿剂。水煎,分两次温服。

2) 针灸:① 基本穴位、配穴(单/双侧)。② 针的规格(长度、直径)。③ 操作手法:旋转,提插,电针……④ 操作时间。

例如陆瘦燕医案某案:

处方:胆俞(泻),双阳纲(泻),阳陵泉(泻),双内关(泻),双足三里(补)。

手法:捻转补泻法。留针10分钟。

(4) 西药。

(5) 日常调护:避风寒、调饮食、畅情志。如心脏病:合理少盐膳食、适量运动、戒烟限酒。哮喘:避免接触过敏原,雾霾天尽量减少户外活动,坚持锻炼。

六、门诊病历的作用

(1) 了解病案质量控制对医疗和患者安全的重要性。

(2) 我们可以向古代及现在的医家学习经验。

(3) 病历能帮助医生与同行间进行交流。病历对医疗、预防、教学、科研、医院管理等都有着重要的作用。

(4) 证明医生的医疗实践:一份良好的病历对医生及患者都是非常有利的。至少40%的医疗过失索赔预防的关键在于病案质量。记载模糊、信息缺失几乎造成了一半的医疗事故案件。医疗记录往往是唯一的真理来源。它们远比记忆更可靠。

七、阅读材料

(1) 病历:书写与保存。

（2）《医学衷中参西录》医案一则。

天津王姓，年三十余，得牙疼病。

病因：商务劳心，又兼连日与友宴饮，遂得斯证。

证候：牙疼甚剧，有碍饮食，夜不能寐，服一切治牙疼之药不效，已迁延二十余日矣。其脉左部如常，而右部弦长，按之有力。

诊断：此阳明胃气不降也。

处方：生赭石一两（轧细），怀牛膝一两，滑石六钱，甘草一钱煎汤服。

效果：将药煎服 1 剂，牙疼立愈，俾按原方再服 1 剂以善其后。

帮助：方书治牙疼未见有用赭石牛膝者，因愚曾病牙疼以二药治愈，后凡遇胃气不降致牙疼者，方中必用此二药。

（3）陆瘦燕医案一则。

邱某，男，64 岁。

初诊（1964 年 8 月 18 日）

1961 年 5 月因腹痛、黄疸反复发作在松江人民医院施行总胆管引流术，术后诊断为慢性胆囊炎、慢性胰腺炎。手术后腹痛发作依旧，每遇饮食不节，即引起上腹部疼痛，平时两胁胀痛，头昏乏力。脉濡细，舌质暗红，苔白腻。甲木犯胃，湿浊中阻，治拟疏泄少阳，化湿和胃。

处方：胆俞（泻），双阳纲（泻），阳陵泉（泻），双内关（泻），双足三里（补）。

手法：捻转补泻，留针 10 分钟。

根据上方，每周针治二次，脘腹隐痛渐减，胃纳亦增。自第七诊后，于原方基础上再加肝俞-，脾俞+。至第十诊时，大便、食欲均已正常，胁痛得除。

八、课后习题

（1）请写出以下病历的主诉

病例 1：我已经几个月不舒服了。做完任何事我都觉得筋疲力尽。我吃不下去饭，体重减轻了 10 千克。

病例 2：前日我乘地铁上班。空调很冷，我只穿 T 恤和短裙。回家后，我感到不舒服，我的肌肉疼痛，关节疼痛，尤其是肩部和背部。

（2）收集现病史：假如你要收集一名水肿患者的现病史，你需要问些什么问题？

参考文献

［1］埃里克·格伦迪宁，罗恩·霍华德.剑桥医学英语［M］.北京：人民邮电出版社，2010.

［2］医学全在线.病历的书写与保存［EB/OL］.［2009 - 12 - 06］. http://www.med126.com/yingyu/2009/159765.shtml.

［3］李冀.方剂学［M］.北京：中国中医药出版社,2012.

Chapter Four

TCM Medical Record Classification and TCM Outpatient Record Writing

TCM outpatient record has the longest history of medical record keeping, maybe the earliest type of medical records we come into contacting with. In retrospect, TCM outpatient record can be divided into three types: verite records, reminiscing records and modern records. In this chapter we will learn the definition, classification and relationship of these three types. Examples of different types may help you better absorb the knowledge. By learning this chapter, you can write a correct complete TCM outpatient modern record.

1. Definition

1.1 Verite records The verite record is written during the clinic consultation. The verite record is known as "An", which was popular in the Qing Dynasty, leaving records acknowledging outpatient visits. The first page is for discussion or comment, which is followed by recording the treatment, generally written as a prescription.

1.2 Reminiscing records Reminiscing records, also regarded as "medical talk", recording the medical diagnosis after registering and reminiscing about all the treatment process, therapeutic effects, and side effects during diagnosis.

1.3 Modern standard formatted records The aims of the medical record are to describe the systematic documentation of a single patient's medical history and care across time within one particular health care provider's jurisdiction. The medical record includes a variety of types of "notes" entered over time by health care professionals, recording observations and administration of drugs and therapies, orders for the administration of drugs and therapies, test results, etc.

Modern TCM doctors write an itemized account of patients' general condition and symptoms, pathology, diagnosis, therapy, prescription, effect, etc., following the western medical records and classification system, so that records are more comprehensive. On this basis, sometimes it is called medical record type basis.

1.4 The Relationship between verite records、reminiscing records and medical records

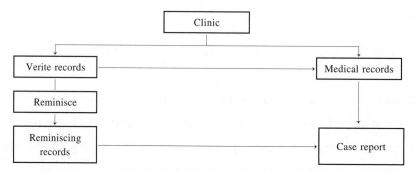

Figure 4 − 1 　The relationship between verite records、reminiscing records and medical records

2. Verite Records

2.1 Characteristics of activity records

2.1.1 　Illness or symptoms record must be real.

2.1.2 　Herbs, dosage and processing projects should faithfully reflect the doctor diagnosis and treatment.

2.2 Famous records 　*Clinical Guidelines Basis*, *in the Late Edition of Commentaries Ye's Records*, *Liu Four Records*, *Ding Gan Ren Records* and *Famous Doctor's Records Essence in the Qing Dynasty*, etc.

2.3 Types of verite record

2.3.1 　First recording the symptoms, next an analysis of etiology and pathogenesis, then the diagnosis and the treatment.

For example:

Symptoms: Mrs. Wang, an old woman, felt chills and fever, vomiting, can neither eat nor drink, abdominal pain, diarrhea 50 − 60 times a day, stool was white and red, tenesmus, thick coating, and shallow tight and quick pulse.

Pathogenesis: Caught the wind evil while late summer prevailing dampness and hot caused hysteresis, damaging of Wei-Qi, and stagnant intestines and stomach.

Diagnosis: anorectic dysentery.

Treatment principle: relieving exterior syndrome, and dredging stagnant.

Decoction:

Jinjie 5 g	Fangfeng 3 g	Douchi 9 g
Bohe 3 g	Banxia 6 g	Zhishi 5 g
Jiegeng 3 g	Chishao 5 g	Shenqu 9 g
Coke Shanzha 9 g	Fresh Ginger 2 slices	Black Tea 3 g
Huoxiang Geng 5 g	Sugeng 5 g	Yushu Pill

From *Ding Gan Ren Records*

2.3.2 First recording the pathogenesis, then symptoms, and finally treatment.

For example: Pathogenesis, The evil from Shao Yang depressed into Jue Yin, and then inversely attack Yang Ming.

Symptom: Alternately felt hot and cold, looked green, vertex and lower abdomen pain.

Treatment principle: Discharging Jue Yin excess, and strengthening spleen and stomach.

Decoction: Zuojin pill and Xiaoyao decoction.

Renshen	Chaihu	Chuanlian
Chenpi	Banxia	Huangqin
Wuyu	Fuling	Gancao

From *Liu four Records*

2.3.3 Records that emphasis the analysis symptoms' reasons, grasping the major cause to get the result.

Lateral thorax pain occurs in spring, stops after spring, which is liver illness. In March spring liver commands, liver Yang is excess, but Yin couldn't follow Yang, so Qi is blocked, then it would cause pain; until summer or autumn liver Yang Qi becomes less, meet yin, so pain stops.

Herbs:

Ejiao	Baishao	Fuling	Danpi
Qiancao	Gancao	using Abalone soup as water to decoction	

From *Liu four Records*

2.3.4 Describe and discuss together with symptoms, cause, etiology, diagnosis and

treatment

Mr. Cai, if talking about illness, you should discuss constitution, shape color and pulse condition first. Because an illness pathogen attacks him from outside. The patient's weak muscle and white skin is Qi deficiency. And Yang deficiency body is apt to be caught dampness and phlegm.

Renshen   Banxia   Fresh Baizhu   Zhishi

Fuling   Fresh Ginger

From *Clinical Guidelines Basis*

3. Reminiscing Records

3.1　Characteristics of reminiscing records　The characteristics of reminiscing records are the diagnosis made and the treatment process used make the curative effect relatively clear. Some records have the acknowledgment of dialectical medication experience, with words more vivid and easy to read. This kind of record is useful to summarize the academic value of medical works or make a deeper impression to experience as academic evidence. Reminiscing records can not only be published, but also be useful in medical works.

3.2　Types of reminiscing record

3.2.1　Simply describe but not or seldom discuss illness treatment process.

Mostly it is doctor's individual experience. Most of these records were developed in the Song, Jin, Yuan, and Ming Dynasty.

Example:

Mr Jin first sweated slightly, aversion to the wind, and his pulse was weak. So the doctor gave him Herba Ephedra (Mahuang). He subsequenly sweated a lot, and had a fever. He also felt palpitations, and could not sleep well at night. He became delirious with muscle twitching and cramp. The doctor gave him a decoction for expelling the wind pathogen. I think this kind of symptom was the mistake of diaphoresis. Zhang Zhongjing once said that if the patient was slightly sweating and had aversion to wind with weak pulse, doctors could not give them Da Qing Long Decoction. If they did, the patient would have muscle twitching and cramp, which was a sign of wrong treatment. We should use Zhen Wu Decoction assisted with Qing Xin Pill. Several days the patient was recovered.

From Records *Pu Ji Ben Shi Decoction*

3. 2.2   A detailed account of the medical process and experiences of differentiation.

Example:

Mr Zhong had abdominal pain for several years. He felt better after he had took Li Zhong Decoction and Si Ni Decoction. However the frequency of pain was irregular, sometimes once a month or twice a month. The pain occurred after he ate cold things, and alleviated after he had pepper and ginger soup. One day he asked me to treat him. His pulse was deep tight and string, and his tongue was white and wet without coating. Slight pain in abdomen when I touched, which would radiate to the waist and hypochondrium. Defecation was scanty and not smooth and the urination was fine. I think the patient's disease was caused by cold stagnation, which should be treated by warming and purgation. However the former treatment only aimed at warming. After the patient took two decoctions of my prescription, he recovered.

Dahuang Fuzi Decoction:

Dahuang   Wufu   Xixin

From Records *Memoirs of Notable Curative Effect*

4. Medical Record Type

4. 1   History of medical record type   After the appearance of *Records of Traditional Chinese and Western Medicine in Combination* written by Zhang Xichun, a famous doctor in Modern times, this form of the medical records became standard and formed the embryonic form of today's medical records.

4. 2   The structure of medical record type

4.2.1   Date and time.

4.2.2   Identification: Including a patient's name, age, occupation, etc.

4.2.3   Chief Complain.

4.2.4   History of present illness.

4.2.5   10 questions: Designed by Zhang Jingyue in the Ming Dynasty, and revised by Chen Xiuyuan in the Qing Dynasty.

First ask hot and cold; Second ask sweat;

Third ask head and body; Forth ask stools and urine;

Fifth ask food and drink; Sixth ask chest;

Seventh ask hearing; Eighth ask thirst;

Ninth ask old disease; Tenth ask cause.

Especially ask the condition of menses for women, delayed, advanced, blocked or flooded.

And for children, ask the past history of measles and chicken pox.

4.2.6　Simple previous and other history and allergy.

4.2.7　Tongue and pulse examination: a. Tongue: Size, color, coating, movement. b. Pulse: Cun-Guan-Chi (bilateral).

4.2.8　Diagnosis: TCM diagnose including name of the disease and differentiation. Western medicine diagnosis.

4.2.9　Treatment/Principle.

4.2.10　Prescription.

4.2.11　Signature.

4.3　Taking a history

4.3.1　What is a medical history: The medical history is information gained by a doctor by asking specific questions, from either of the patient or of other people who know the person and who can give suitable information, with the aim of obtaining information useful in formulating a diagnosis and providing medical care to the patient.

4.3.2　How to write the chief complaint: The chief complaint is the main reason or one of the most obvious symptoms (signs, properties) the patient presents with and its duration. The first diagnosis corresponds to the chief complaint. The chief complain should be written in the patient's words with no more than 20 Chinese characters. For example "chest pain" rather than "angina".

When doctors ask patients' symptoms, they use their way to express their pain or uncomfortable. Doctors should extract the information from the patient's own words.

For example:

I was well until a few months ago. In the beginning of August (now in October), I just felt off-color and a bit tired. But lately I've been feeling completely worn out at the end of the day. I am not eating any more like usual but I have put on nine kilos in the last year. My motions are hard and my hair has started to fall out.

Chief complaint: Fatigue has gradually increased for 3 months, with hair loss.

Other ways to write chief complain (Table 4 - 1):

Table 4 - 1 Comparison of expressing the main complaint

Correct Expression	Wrong Expression
Chest pain for 2 hours	The patient felt pain in chest for 2 hours
Two-day history of (sustained/fluctuant) fever	39℃ , 2 days
Nausea and vomiting of three days' duration	The patient felt nausea at first and then he vomited a lot gastric content day after day for nearly three days
Headache 1 month in duration	The patient said she had a headache for a month

4.3.3　How to collect information of history of present illness: The history of present illness is a more detailed description of the patient's main complaint. It is the most important structural element of the medical history. Usually doctors may collect information like: causative factors, sites, character, duration, severity, frequency, timing, aggravating factors, relieving factors, associated features, etc. It also includes details about the previous clinical experience, like when, which hospital, diagnoses, tests, treatments, effect, related negative symptoms, etc. The related negative symptoms are also important. Sometimes two diseases have similar signs and symptoms. Doctors can make differential diagnosis according to the important negative symptoms.

For example, in respect to pain (Table 4 - 2):

Table 4 - 2 Tipical question of pain

Feature	Typical question
Main site	Where does it hurt
Radiation	Does it go anywhere else
Character	Can you describe the pain (burning, crushing, gnawing, gripping, sharp, stabbing, stinging, throbbing)
Precipitating factors	Does anything bring them on
Time of onset	When do they stop
Frequency	How often do you get them
Aggravating factors	Does anything make them worse
Relieving factors	Does anything make them better
Associated features	Do you feel anything else wrong when it's there? Have you any other problems related to the pain
Duration	How long do they last
Severity	How bad is it

Doctors should pay attention to some other problems which may be related and relevant to the disease:

4.3.3.1 Congenital factors: Premature birth, birth injury, congenital malformation, genetic metabolic diseases.

4.3.3.2 Emotional stimulation: Changing the environment, the lack of care or accompany, emotional problem.

4.3.3.3 Unexpected factors: Accidental injury, fall from the high place, fall into the water, burns, foreign body inhalation.

4.3.3.4 Other factors: Environment (fog, smoking, decoration), food (hormones).

For example: a. Runny nose after the cold. b. Abdominal pain and diarrhea due to eating unclean food. c. Cough and asthma after his father's smoking.

4.3.4 How to document a previous history, family history, drug history including allergies: Previous history includes eczema, asthma, malnutrition, rickets and other medical history. Doctors also need to write family history about asthma, allergic diseases and metabolic diseases and allergies including drugs and food. For children, doctors should record personal history including birth history, feeding history, growth and development history and vaccination history.

4.3.5 How to document tongue inspection: Tongue is a microcosm of the entire body and will reflect its excesses and deficiencies. Shape, color, coating and texture of the tongue can indicate digestive issues and body imbalances.

The gold standard: A normal healthy tongue is pink in color with light white tongue coating, and is proportionate in size to the mouth. The neonatal tongue is red without coating. Eating and medicine taken will influence the tongue inspection, so the tongue need to be cleaned by gargling and should be observed in natural light. Different parts of the tongue correspond to different organs (Figure 4 - 2、Figure 4 - 3).

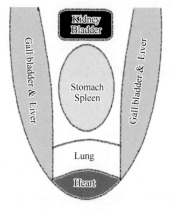

Figure 4 - 2　Tongue

4.3.5.1 Tongue appearance: a. Fat: Yang deficiency. b. Dark purple: stasis. c. Pale: Qi and blood deficiency. d. Scarlet: heat penetrating the blood.

4.3.5.2 Presence of fur a. Yellow and greasy: damp heat. b. Exfoliative: Yin deficiency.

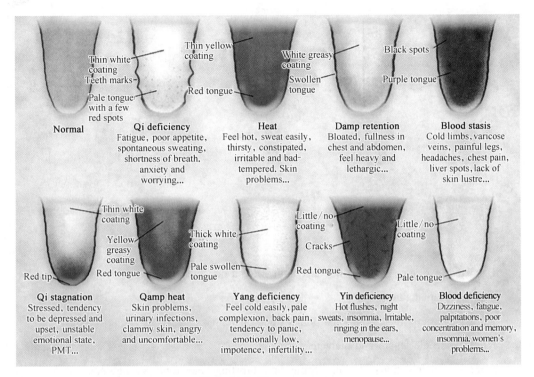

Figure 4 - 3　Tongue appearance

5. How to Write A Formal Prescription

5. 1　Herbal treatment　(including the name of herbs, dosage and how to take the decoction). Chief — The main drugs/method for primary symptom or disease. Deputy — To play a role of auxiliary medicine. Assistant — To treat side symptoms or avoid drug side effects. Envoy — To guide the drugs to the lesions, or harmonize drugs.

5. 2　Other treatments　Acupuncture, moxibustion, cupping, Traditional Chinese Medicine fumigation, Daoyin (Baduanjin, Wuqinxi) (Figure 4 - 4).

Including the frequency of treatment, the time of treatment (Zi Wu Liu Zhu: midnight-midday ebb flow theory).

5. 3　Format

5. 3.1　Herbal

Herbal A ＿＿ g　Herbal B ＿＿ g　Herbal C ＿＿ g　Herbal D ＿＿ g

Herbal E ＿＿ g　Herbal F ＿＿ g　Herbal G ＿＿ g　Herbal H ＿＿ g

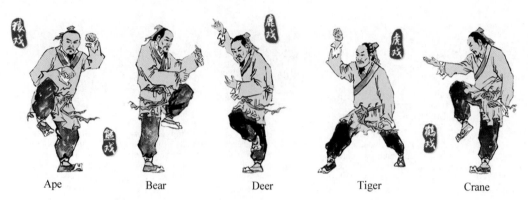

| Ape | Bear | Deer | Tiger | Crane |

Figure 4 – 4   Wuqinxi

…… X ____ dosages

Decocted in water, and take the decoction twice a day.

5. 3.2   Acupuncture

5.3.2.1   basic points, additional points (uni/bilateral).

5.3.2.2   needle length and diameter.

5.3.2.3   manipulation: twirling, lifting and thrusting, electronic needle, etc.

5.3.2.4   duration time

5.3.2.5   frequency of treatment

For example:

Prescription: Danshu (reducing), Yanggang (bilateral, reducing), Yanglingquan (reducing), Neiguan (bilateral, reducing), Zusanli (bilateral, reinforcing)

Manipulation: reinforcing or reducing by twirling or rotating the needle with needle retaining for 10 minutes.

From Lu Shouyan's medical records

5. 4   Western medicine

5. 5   Daily health-care recommendation

Avoiding getting cold, adjusting diet and maintaining good mood.

For example:

5.5.1   Heart disease — having low-salt and balanced diet, having moderate exercise, quitting smoking and limiting alcohol.

5.5.2   Asthma — avoiding exposure to allergen, having indoor activity during haze days, having physical exercises.

6. Function and General Tips

6.1 Understand the importance of medical records in quality control of health care and patient's safety.

6.2 Learn from the ancient or current doctors' experience through TCM records.

6.3 The medical record helps doctors communicate among the peer   The medical records play vital role in medical treatments, prevention, teaching, scientific researches, hospital administration and so on.

6.4 Find the evidence to prove doctors' medical practice   A good medical record serves the interests of the medical practitioner as well as his patients. The key to defensibility of at least 40% of all medical negligence claims rests with the quality of the medical records. Illegibility, inadequacy or absence dooms almost half of medical negligence cases. Medical records are often the only source of truth. They are likely to be far more reliable than memory.

7. Reading Materials

7. 1 Medical records   Making and Retaining.

7. 2 A medical record selected from *Records of Traditional Chinese and Western Medicine in Combination*   Mr. Wang, who was in his thirties, lived in Tianjin, got the toothache.

Etiology: Busy business and uncontrolled party with drinking without restraint.

Symptom: A serious toothache affected appetite, caused insomnia, taking any medicine for treating did not have a good curative effect, which had tormented the patient for more than 20 days.

Pulse condition: Normal pulse on the left hand, wiry, powerful and long on the other.

Diagnosis: Undescending of gastric Qi.

Prescription: Sheng Zheshi(1 ounce, powder-like)   Huai Niuxi(1 ounce)   Huashi(0.6 ounce)   Gancao(0.1 ounce).

Decocted in water.

Curative effect: Quickly recovered after a dose, continued to one more dose to consolidate efficacy.

Tips: In medical records before, no one used Sheng Zheshi and Huai Niuxi for toothache treating, but after I cured my own toothache by these two herbs accidently, I used to treat this kind of disease the same way.

7.3　An acupuncture medical record selected from *Lu Shouyan's Record*　Mr Qiu, male, 64 years old, First visit: 1964.8.18

In May 1961, Mr Qiu had choledochus drainage in Songjiang Hosptial because of abdominal pain and jaundice recurrence. Postoperative diagnosis were chronic cholecystitis and chronic pancreatitis. However the pain reoccurred when he ate a lot. He usually felt pain in lateral thorax, dizzy and fatigue. Pulse: small and soft pulse. Tongue: tongue quality was dark red and coating was white and greasy. Liver Qi invading stomach caused dampness obstructing the middle.

Treating principle: Soothing liver Qi, dissipating dampness and strengthening stomach.

Prescription: BL19 Danshu (reducing), BLA8 Shuang Yanggang (reducing), GB34 Yang Lingquan(reducing),P6 Shuang Neiguan(reducing),ST36 Shuang Zusanli(reinforcing)

Manipulation: Reinforcing-reducing method by twirling. Needle left for 10 minutes.

Curative effect: According to this method twice a week, patient's abdominal pain was released and he had a good appetite ... After the 7th visit BL18 and BL 20 were added. After 10th visit, the patient's appetite and feces were normal, with lateral thorax pain released.

8. Homework

Homework 1　Please write the chief complain of the following cases:

Case 1: I haven't been myself for several months now. I feel completely worn out after doing anything. I've been off my food and I've lost ten kilos in weight.

Case 2: I went to work by underground the day before yesterday. The air conditioner was very cold, and I just wore T-shirt and short skirt. When I went back home, I felt unwell. I had pain in muscles and also pain in joints, especially in shoulders and back.

Homework 2　Collecting history of present history: If you are a doctor collecting a history of edema patient's present history, what questions would you ask?

References

[1] Eric HG, Ron H. Professional English in use medicine[M]. Beijing: Posts & Telecom Press, 2010.

［2］ Medical Records：Making and Retaining Them［EB/OL］. ［2009 - 12 - 06］. http：//www. med126.com/yingyu/2009/159765.shtml.

［3］ Li J. Formulas of Chinese Medicine［M］. Beijing：China Press of Traditional Chinese Medicine, 2012.

第五章　专科门诊病历书写

除了普通门诊病案书写外,我们在临床实践中还会遇到各种类型的专科门诊病案书写。在第四章中,我们学习了普通门诊病历的基本结构。在此基础上,门诊各专科病案对病史收集、体格检查、处方书写的要求各有不同。本章将以儿科、妇科、针灸为例进行讲解。

一、定义

门诊病历是在诊疗过程中(如检查、诊断、治疗)对疾病发生、发展、预后结果的过程的记录,是门诊实践的重要总结,在疾病治疗、疾病预防、科学研究以及医疗管理方面都起到非常重要的作用。

二、一般门诊病历的基本结构框架

1. 门诊病历本封面　包括患者姓名、性别、年龄、婚育、职业、联系电话、地址、保险等基本信息。

2. 门诊病历内容

(1)主诉:患者最痛苦的症状体征及其持续时间。

(2)病史:它是对于患者自发病以来的全过程,即发生、发展、预后等的描述。包括:起病时间、诱因、主要症状、检查和治疗,家族史,既往史,婚育史,个人生活史(是否吸烟或饮酒)。

(3)体格检查:记录主要的阳性体征及有助于鉴别诊断的阴性体征。

中医检查应特别注意舌象及脉象的描述。

(4)辅助检查:患者需要做的相关检查(如血的检验、超声及放射性检查等),以帮助医生诊断疾病。

（5）初步诊断：应同时包括中医诊断与西医诊断。

（6）治疗：应同时包括所开具的所有药物以及服药方法。

（7）临床建议应视具体情况而调整。如：

1）特殊患者，如高血压病患者饮食应清淡。

2）痛经患者少食寒凉之物。

3）胃病患者应少食辛辣刺激。

4）糖尿病患者宜少食甜食，多运动。

5）肺病患者避免感冒等。

一般情况多建议三餐合理膳食；春捂秋冻；懂得宣泄、控制情绪；避风寒、畅情志；饮食规律、常运动等。

（8）接诊医生签名及日期（若为急诊就诊，时间需精确至分钟）。

三、专科门诊病历书写

门诊病历书写除了上述通用书写规范，儿科、妇科、针灸科有特殊的书写要求。

1. 儿科门诊病历

（1）鉴于新生儿和婴幼儿特殊的生理特点，儿科门诊医生还需特别注意以下几点：出生史、喂养史、生长发育史、接种史，刻下饮食、二便，哺乳期的母亲饮食状况。

1）出生史：① 分娩时的胎龄，即足月或早产。② 是否有呼吸暂停。③ 是否难产。④ 母亲怀孕时的营养及健康状况。

2）喂养史：① 喂养方式及辅食，断奶时间。② 饮食习惯。③ 是否甜、烫、辣、腻。④ 是否含肉或蔬菜。⑤ 是否含鸡蛋或牛奶。⑥ 烫或凉。⑦ 食欲状况。

3）生长发育史：① 6 月龄，坐。② 8 月龄，爬。③ 10 月龄，走。④ 18 月龄，跑。⑤ 24 月龄，跳。⑥ 语言。⑦ 萌牙时间。⑧ 体重及身高生长状况。

4）接种史：① 按照标准流程的接种时间。② 荨麻疹疫苗。③ 流感疫苗。④ 肺炎疫苗。

（2）儿科中的"十问歌"（"十问歌"为一首综合中医问诊要点的歌赋，因其包含 10 句问诊内容，被称为"十问歌"）。

1）问寒热：医生要区分寒证（恶寒）、热证（恶热）、里热及消化不良（手足心热）。

2）问汗：医生需要询问患者发汗的原因，如天气炎热，穿衣过多，饮热食或热水，剧烈运动等。还需要了解汗量、出汗位置及出汗时间，并需注意孩子比成年人更容易出汗。如：

① 自汗：白天出汗，轻微运动会出汗更多（气虚）。② 盗汗：睡时汗出，醒来汗止（阴虚）。③ 冷汗（阳虚）。

3）问头身：成年人和年龄较大的儿童可以辨别头痛、头晕和身体其他部位的疼痛和不适。但对于幼儿来说，你会发现他们很难描述自己的症状。医生则需要依靠更密切的观察加以诊断。例如，头痛伴呕吐、高热和抽搐提示婴儿急性惊厥。

4）问大便：医生应留意便量、特征、颜色及气味。如：① 稀便+白色血块：牛奶或食物消化不良。② 味臭（臭鸡蛋样）+腹泻/腹痛：消化不良。③ 长期腹泻：气阴两虚。④ 便秘：热盛，气滞，阴虚，气虚。⑤ 便黄，水样，味臭且次数多：发热伴呕吐。

5）问小便：医生需询问尿量及颜色。尿量与饮水量及汗量有关。如：① 黄短赤：下焦湿热，或心火下移小肠。② 尿血鲜红：热伤脉络。③ 粉红尿：气不摄血。④ 尿浊：脾虚。⑤ 遗尿：肾虚。

6）问饮食：需询问饮食的细节，包括食物和饮水。医生需要询问食欲及饮水量。如：食欲不振伴疲乏，脾虚；多饮少食，舌干便秘，胃阴虚。

7）问睡眠：① 年龄越小，睡眠时间越长。② 夜啼：腹痛或受惊。③ 睡中露睛：脾虚。④ 嗜睡：痰蒙清窍。

8）望面部：通常患儿太小，无法描述自身的症状。医生需要观察面部和肤色来收集信息（图5－1）。

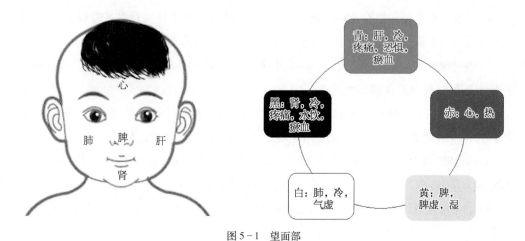

图5－1 望面部

（3）特殊查体，如小儿指纹。示指近虎口第一节为风关，第二节为气关，第三节为命关。红紫分寒热，淡滞定虚实。指纹分别显现于风、气、命三关甚至透关射甲说明病情进展。

（4）特殊治疗，如小儿贴敷治疗，须写明药味、穴位、贴服时间、注意事项。如治疗期间一般禁食生冷、油腻、辛辣食物。耳穴治疗须写明穴位及按揉时间。如小儿脾虚泄泻，肉豆蔻、吴茱萸、小茴香各 6 克,研成粉末,加入葱白,捣烂如泥状,敷于肚脐,每日 2 次,每次 3 小时,连用 7 日为 1 个疗程。将王不留行籽贴于胃、大肠耳部穴位处,每日 3 次,每次按压 2 分钟,直至耳部变红为度。

2. **妇科门诊病历书写** 见表 5 - 1。

表 5 - 1 妇科门诊病历内容

项 目	内 容
月经	日期、量、色(红/紫/褐)、血块、持续时间、其他症状(头痛、腹泻、便秘、呕吐等)
带下	量、色、血、质地(稀薄/黏稠)
妊娠状态	次数、何时/流产次数和时间、方式
生产	次数、何时、方式(人工流产或药物流产)

经期史、婚孕史必须在妇科记录中提及。

妇科病历书写有特殊的表述方法,如"1 - 0 - 1 - 1""$G_2P_1L_1A_1$""14 7/28, LMP April 3rd, 2017."。

"1 - 0 - 1 - 1"表示"足月产-早产-流产-存活"。

"$G_0P_0L_0A_0$"表示"妊娠;生产;存活;流产"。

"14 7/28, LMP:April 3rd, 2017."表示"初次来潮 14 岁;月经周期 28 日,每次 7 日,末次月经 2017 年 4 月 3 日"。

3. **中医外科手术病历书写**

(1) 局部区域:皮肤颜色,皮温,肿块高度,肿块范围,肿块硬度,脓液等变化。

(2) 一般情况:是否发热、恶寒、口干、口渴、尿少、便秘、舌红、苔黄、脉快等。例如:感染部位皮肤肿胀,呈鲜红色,有灼痛感,边缘清晰。无化脓,但伴有感冒、发热和头痛。直肠指诊(DRE)是中医四诊触诊的一种检查方法,是临床表现与中医临床模式相结合的一种检查方法,是一种极其有效的鉴别方法。如湿热瘀阻型患者除了主要表现为小便黄或微红、尿道分泌物白浊、舌苔黄腻、脉滑且数,指诊检查显示腺体肿大、按压后排出大量黏稠前列腺液,前列腺柔软。

4. **针灸门诊病历书写** 在门诊,针灸医生需要在治疗一栏明确写清穴位、手法、留针时间及其他治疗方法,如艾灸、电针、拔罐等。治疗频次也需注明。

5. **膏方门诊病历书写** 在中医理论中,膏方是一种高营养、高疗效、防治作用强的中成药。膏方是以大型复方汤剂为基础,根据患者不同体质及临床表现配制而成的浓稠膏状或冷冻制剂。

(1) 病史、刻下症、舌苔脉象。

(2) 药物及剂量(一般四味药一行,药味总共在 40~60 味)。

（3）服用方法及注意事项。

除上述一般门诊病历外,服药注意事项也应注明。

如空腹服:可以使药物迅速入肠,并且保持较高浓度而迅速发挥药效。

饭前服:一般在饭前 30~60 分钟时服药。病情较轻,饭前服药可使药物更快发挥作用。

饭后服:一般在饭后 15~30 分钟时服药。可以使药物的效果保持更长时间。

睡前服:一般在睡前 15~30 分钟时服用。镇静安眠的药物宜睡前服。

四、课后习题

根据以下信息,请尝试写三个完整的门诊病历。

病例 1:6 个月前,李梅(23 岁,大学生)为准备考试熬夜 1 周,随后出现月经推迟,至今没来。她经常感到小腹疼痛,像针刺,并且易发怒。她从未在外院就诊过,也没擅自服用过任何药物。早早孕显示未孕。每日饮食、排便规律,睡眠不佳,夜梦多。她未婚未育,末次月经时间 2016 年 10 月 1 日。未避孕,从未流产,带下正常。既往没有患过传染病,否认手术史、过敏史。舌紫黯,脉涩。

病例 2:2 日前,李军(9 个月大)突发咳嗽、流涕、有痰,昨日发热,体温最高 38.5℃。他出生在 2016 年 3 月。第一胎,顺产,出生时体重 3 千克。孩子妈妈的母乳很少,喂养主要以奶粉为主。4 个月时,加米汤、蒸蛋等辅食,5 个月时,加饼干、苹果泥等辅食。7 个月时会坐,现在能在帮助下站立,但还不会走。6 个月时曾患感冒。没有得过麻疹和水痘。出生 1 周时接种卡介苗,8 个月时接种百白破。舌红苔薄白,脉浮数。

病例 3:王某,23 岁,女性。腰背部位疼痛反复长达 1 年,每遇劳累后、阴雨天加重。3 日前雨后突觉腰痛加重。未婚未育。既往体健。舌淡苔白,脉滑。

参考文献

[1] 张戈.规范书写病历是减少医疗纠纷的重要一环[J].中国医学伦理学,2003,16(5):37.

[2] 张建伟.如何指导实习生书写中医妇科病历[J].中国医案,2008,9(7):48-49.

[3] 吴健,武士锋,杨洪涛.膏方在内科疾病治疗中的应用概况[J].中华中医药杂志,2013,28(9):2690-2693.

Chapter Five

Specialized Outpatient Record Writing

In addition to the general outpatient medical record writing, we will also encounter various types of specialized outpatient medical record writing in clinical practice. In chapter 4, we have learned the basic structure of general outpatient medical records. On this basis, the requirements of medical history collection, physical examination and prescription writing are different from each specialized outpatient record. This chapter will take pediatrics, gynecology, acupuncture and moxibustion as examples.

1. Definition

Outpatient medical record is medical information relating to the disease's onset, development and outcome of the patient in conjunction with medical actions such as inspection, diagnosis and treatment process. Outpatient medical record is the summary of the clinical practice work. It has an important role in medical treatment, disease prevention, scientific research, and hospital management.

2. The Structure of General Outpatient Record Writing

2.1 **Outpatient record note cover**   The clinical notes include the patient's name, gender, age, marital status, occupation, contact details, address, health insurance, etc.

2.2 Medical records should further include

2.2.1   Chief complaint, namely the patient's most painful symptoms or signs, and its duration.

2.2.2   Medical history that describes the whole course of the illness after the onset, namely the occurrence, development, etc. The medical record should include: the starting time of the illness, causes prognosis, main symptoms, examination and treatment, family history, previous history, marital status history, and the social history (including smoking or drinking).

2.2.3　Physical examination refers to the main positive body signs and negative signs which can help make differences from other diseases. Particular attention should be made in TCM examination to describe the tongue and pulse.

2.2.4　Auxiliary examination include any pertinent examinations patients need to help doctors make the diagnosis, such as blood tests, ultrasound and radiological examination.

2.2.5　Early diagnosis include both the TCM and the WM diagnosis.

2.2.6　Treatment should describe all the medication prescribed and the instructions about how to take medicine.

2.2.7　Lifestyle advice will vary according to the condition. Thus, for example:

2.2.7.1　Special patients, such as those with high blood pressure should have a light diet.

2.2.7.2　Patients with dysmenorrhea will eat less cold food.

2.2.7.3　Patients with stomach disease eat less spicy food.

2.2.7.4　People with diabetes should eat less sugar and exercise more.

2.2.7.5　Patients with lung disease are away from colds with regular lifestyle.

In general, advice is given to eat reasonable meals; "keep warm in spring and cool in autumn"; express and control emotion reasonably; avoid wind chill, be happy, eat regularly, and perform regular exercise.

2.2.8　Physician signature and date (if it is an emergency record, that should be accurate to the minute).

3. The Specialized Outpatient Record

In addition to the general outpatient medical record writing standards above, pediatrics, gynecology, acupuncture clinic outpatient record writings have their special academic writing style.

3.1　Pediatrics record writing

3.1.1　In view of the infants and young children's special physiological characteristics, outpatient doctors also need to get the following information: birth history, history of feeding, the development of children and history of immunization, diet at present, stool and urination, the diet of a breastfeeding mother.

3.1.1.1　Birth history, for example: Gestational age at delivery, i. e. full-term or premature, apnea, dystocia, mother's nutrition and health during pregnancy.

3.1.1.2　Feeding history, for example: Feeding patterns and supplemental food, weaning time. Eating habits. Sweet, hot, spicy, greasy. Meat or vegetable. Eggs or milk. Hot or cold. Appetite.

3.1.1.3　Growth and developmental history, for example: 6 months old — sitting. 8 months old — crawling. 10 months old — standing. 12 months old — walking. 18 months old — running. 24 month old — jumping. Language. Teeth eruption time. Weight and length growth.

3.1.1.4　Vaccination history, for example: Timing according to standard schedule. Measles vaccine. Influenza vaccine. Pneumonia vaccine.

3. 1.2　"Ten questions songs" in pediatrics(Ten questions songs is a song that integrates the main points of TCM consultation, and it contains ten consultation questions, so it is called "ten questions songs").

3.1.2.1　Ask about the cold and heat　Doctors need to distinguish cold syndrome (aversion to cold), heat syndrome (aversion heat) and heat inside or indigestion (feverish sensation in palm and foot).

3.1.2.2　Ask about sweating　Doctors need to ask patients causing factors such as hot weather, too thick coats, eating hot food or water and heavy movement. Doctors also need to know quantity, location and time, and notice that children are easier to sweat than adult.

For example:

3.1.2.2.1　Spontaneous sweating　Sweat in the daytime and sweat more with slight movement (Qi deficiency).

3.1. 2. 2. 2　Night sweating　Sweat at sleep time and stop when waking up (Yin deficiency).

3.1.2.2.3　Cold sweating (Yang deficiency)

3.1.2.3　Ask about head and body symptomatology: Adults and older children can tell a headache, dizziness and other parts of the body pain and discomfort. For children, you may find it more difficult to describe their symptoms. Doctors need to rely more on close observation. For example, headache with vomiting, high fever and convulsion are suggestive of acute infantile convulsion.

3.1.2.4　Ask of the characteristics of the stool：Doctors collect information about quantity, character, color and smell.

For example：

3.1.2.4.1　Thin stool + white clot　Dyspepsia of milk or food.

3.1.2.4.2　Smelly (like rotten eggs) + diarrhea/abdominal pain　Indigestion.

3.1.2.4.3　Diarrhea for a long time　Qi and Yin deficiency.

3.1.2.4.4　Constipation　Excessive heat, Qi stagnation, Yin deficiency, Qi deficiency.

3.1.2.4.5　Yellow, watery, smelly and frequent　fever with vomiting.

3.1.2.5　Ask about the characteristics of the urine　Doctors need to ask quantity and color. The quantity of the urine relates with the drink and sweat.

For example：

3.1.2.5.1　Yellow, dark and short urine　Damp-heat of lower-Jiao, or heart heat transfer into the small intestine

3.1.2.5.2　Fresh red urine　Heat damage the collaterals.

3.1.2.5.3　Pink urine　Qi cannot control blood.

3.1.2.5.4　Turbid urine　Spleen deficiency.

3.1.2.5.5　Enuresis　Kidney deficiency.

3.1.2.6　Ask for details about the diet, including both food and drink　Doctors need to ask about the appetite and the quantity of fluids taken.

For example：

3.1.2.6.1　Loss of appetite with fatigue　Spleen deficiency.

3.1.2.6.2　Drinking more water and eating less food combined with a dry tongue and constipation　Stomach Yin deficiency.

3.1.2.7　Ask about sleeping pattern：

3.1.2.7.1　The younger the children are, the longer the sleep is.

3.1.2.7.2　Crying at night　Abdominal pain or scared.

3.1.2.7.3　Sleeping with eyelid unclosed　Spleen deficiency.

3.1.2.7.4　Drowsiness　Sputum cover the Qingqiao(the upper orifices or sense organs of the head).

3.1.2.8　Observe the face　Usually children are too young to describe their symptoms. Doctors need to observe the face and complexion to collect information (Figure 5 - 1).

3.1.3　Special check, such as the child's fingerprint　The first section of the index finger

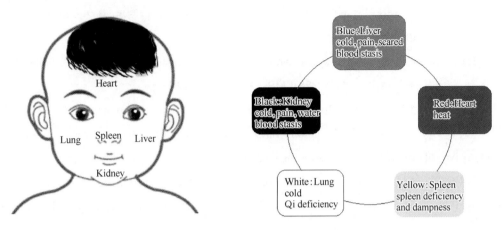

Figure 5 − 1   observe the face

is the wind (Feng Guan), the second is the Qi (Qi Guan), and the third is the life (Ming Guan). If the fingerprint is red, this represents the cold; if purple it represents heat. A sparse fingerprint represents deficiency syndrome; A dense fingerprint represents excessive syndrome. The fingerprints are shown in the wind, Qi, and life, and finally through the fingernail, which represents the progress of the disease.

3. 1.4   Special observations relating to the management, such as children sticking to the treatment, which must be noted in detail with ingredients, acupoint time, and attention such as no cold, greasy and spicy food. The ear acupoint treatment should include the ear acupoint name and massage time. An example of a management record would in the case of infant diarrhea (spleen deficiency syndrome) be: Rou Doukou, Wu Zhuyu, Xiao Huixiang each 6 g grinded into powder, add scallions, mash them to mud, and apply to the navel twice a day, every time for 3 h, 7 days for a course of treatment. Place the seed in the ear acupoint of the stomach and large intestine, and rub it three times a day for two minutes, until the ear becomes red.

3. 2   Gynecology record writing   As show in Table 5 − 1.

Table 5 − 1   Gynecology record writing

Itein	Content
Menstruation	Date, quantity, color (red/purple/brown …), presence of blood clots, duration, other symptoms (headache/diarrhea/constipation/emesis, etc)
Leucorrhea	quantity、color、blood、texture (thin/sticky)
Gestation	times、when、abortion times or miscarriges way
Pregnancy	times、when、way (operation or natural birth)

"Menstrual history" and "Marriage and Pregnancy history" must be mentioned in gynecology records.

There are special standard ways to write gynecology outpatient records. For example: "1 − 0 − 1 − 1" or "$G_2P_1L_1A_1$" or "14 7/28 LMP: April 3rd, 2017."

"1 − 0 − 1 − 1" refers to "full term birth − premature delivery − abortion − live birth".

"$G_0P_0L_0A_0$" refers to: Gestation (times); Pregnancy (premature delivery or full-term birth); Live; Abortion (times, operation or medicine).

"14 7/28, LMP: April 3rd, 2017." Refers to: First menstruation at 14 years of age; menstrual circle is 28 days; each time lasting for 7 days; last menstrual period on April 3rd, 2017.

3.3 Surgery of TCM record writing

Local zone: Change of skin color, skin temperature, height of tumefaction, scope of tumefaction, hardness of tumefaction, change of pus.

General condition: fever, aversion to cold, dry mouth, thirst, scanty urine, constipation, red tongue, yellowish coating, rapid pulse, etc.

For example: Tumefaction in fresh red color, with burning pain and clear margin present in the skin of the infected area. There is no suppuration but associated with cold, fever and headache.

Digital rectal examination (DRE) is a palpation examination method of the TCM Four Examination, which is a combining clinical manifestation with TCM clinical pattern, a particularly useful method in guiding pattern discrimination. For example, besides the main clinical manifestations of patient with the Damp-heat stasis obstruction pattern, yellow or reddish urine, white turbid urethral discharge, red tongue with slimy yellow coating, rolling and rapid pulse, the DRE findings are enlarged gland, large volume of viscous prostatic fluid is emitted after massage, soft prostate after pressing.

3.4 Acupuncture record writing

In the clinic, doctors need to write clearly on "treatment": acupuncture points, techniques, retaining needle time and some other special treatments, such as moxibustion, electric acupuncture, cupping, etc. It is essential to record the frequency of treatment.

3.5 Gao Fang (herbal extract paste)

In the theory of TCM, Gao Fang prescription is a kind of patent medicine with high nutrition, nourishment, treatment and prevention function. It is a thick semi-liquid or frozen formulation based on large-scale compound decoction, which is established according to different constitutions and clinical manifestations of human beings.

3.5.1   Medical history of Gao Fang; manifestation at present; tongue and pulse condition.

3.5.2   Medicine and dose(four herbal names a line, a total of 40－60 herbs).

3.5.3   Attention of taking medicine   In addition to the above general outpatient medical records, the attention of taking medicine should be noted for the precautions. Thus, if taken on an empty stomach, the drug can quickly be into the intestine and remain in high concentration.

Before meals: usually take the medicine 30 to 60 minutes before the meal. The disease is in the lower focus, taking the medicine before meals can make the medicine exert its effect quicker.

After meals: usually take the medicine 15 to 30 minutes after the meal which can make the drug effect stays longer.

Before bed: generally take the medication 15 to 30 minutes before bed. This is advisable for the sleeping medicine.

4. Homework

There are three clinic cases, try to write records according to the information given from the form.

Case 1: 6 months ago, after staying up late for one week for preparing exams, Li Mei's (female, 23 years old, college student) menstruation did not come until now. She often feels abdominal pain, like a needle stabbing, and gets angry very easily. She has not seen a doctor before, and has not taken any medication. Yesterday she took the pregnancy test and that was negative. Normal bowel evacuation, normal diet, not sleeping well, and easily get dreams. She has not been married, last menstruation date: 2016.10.1, no contraception, no abortion and normal leucorrhea. No communicable disease history, no surgery and no allergic history. Her tongue is dark purple, the pulse is uneven.

Case 2: 2 days ago, Li Jun, a nine months old boy, suddenly got a running nose, cough and sputum. Yesterday he developed a fever, the highest temperature being 38.5℃. He was born on March 3, 2016 in hospital, full-term natural labor. His birth weight was 3 kg. His mother's breast milk was scanty, so he was fed mainly with milk powder. When he was four months old, his mother added rice water and steamed eggs to his diet. When he was five months old, his mother added food porridge, biscuits and apple puree to his diet. When he was 7 months old he could sit. Now he can stand up with help, but he still cannot move. When he was six months old, he had cold. No history of measles and chicken pox infection.

1 week after his birth, he was given BCG vaccination, and 8 months after his birth he took the DPT vaccine. His tongue is red with thin and white coating, with floating rapid pulse.

Case 3: Wan Min, a 23-year-old lady, repeatedly felt back pain over the last 1 year. She reported that the pain got worse when she was tired or during rainy days. Three days ago after hard and continuing rain, the pain got worse again. Unmarried and childless. Her tongue is pale with white coating, with smooth pulse.

References

[1] Zhang G. Writing medical records regularly is an important part of reducing medical dispute[J]. Chinese Medical Ethics, 2003, 16(5): 37.

[2] Zhang J. How to instruct interns to write TCM gynecological medical records[J]. Chinese Medical Record, 2008, 9(7): 48-49.

[3] Wu J, Wu S F, Yang H T. Review of application on medical diseases of herbal pastes[J]. China Journal of Traditional Chinese Medicine and Pharmacy, 2013, 28(9): 2690-2693.

第六章 中医住院病历书写

这章节将分为以下几部分进行介绍：中医住院病历书写的概念、中医病历书写的法规及指南、中医住院病历书写的格式、中医住院病历书写的要求、一般注意事项、中医住院病历的作用、建议阅读材料和练习题。

一、中医住院病历书写的概念

病历是描述医务人员在权利管辖范围内对一个患者的病史和治疗的系统记录。病历是医疗、教学、科研工作的第一手资料。同时，病历也是医疗质量评估与医院管理决策的重要依据和办理医疗保险以及处理医疗纠纷事故的原始证据。写病历的水准也是衡量一个医生业务水平的重要指标。因此，病历书写是十分重要的。

病历分为门诊病历和住院病历两部分。住院病历书写是临床医生必须掌握的基本功。通过书写住院病历，可以规范医生采集病史及体格检查，加强医生与患者交流沟通的能力，训练其临床诊断及鉴别诊断的思维，并能培养用综合动态分析患者病情、调整治疗方案的能力。

中医有着自己的理论体系和辨治特点。它是以"证"为基准，诊断、治疗必须观病形、测病因，即通过外形、感觉症、征的表现，以测其内在的病情、病机，更从发生、发展的复杂变化来分析病因、病位、病性和机制。它不仅需要疾病的发生、发展及演变的详细病程记录，还需要对疾病的诊断、治疗及疗效的完整诊疗经过加以记录。所以，中医住院病历有其独特之处，除了西医的病史采集、体格检查外，还需要详细记录患者的四诊信息，并进行归纳、分析，体现辨证思维过程，从而进行中医疾病诊断及证候诊断，制定中医治疗方案。因此，一份好的中医住院病历，既要有疾病发生、病变表现、发展转归的详实情况，也要有贯穿医生的审因测机、辨证论治、组方遣药、疗效变化的实践经过。

主要住院病程记录包括：入院病程记录、首次病程记录、主治医师首次查房记录、主任医师首次查房记录、病程记录。

二、中医住院病历书写的格式

中医住院病历书写的格式要点包括准确性、及时性、完整性、一致性。

一份完整的中医住院病历能体现三级查房制度,应该依序包括以下内容。

(一) 首次病程记录

1. 患者基本信息 患者姓名、年龄、性别、民族、国籍、家庭地址、职业、婚姻状况、入院日期、记录日期、病史申述者、医疗保险情况以及联系电话。

2. 主诉 就诊最主要的原因或最明显的症状或(和)体征、性质,以及持续时间。询问患者主诉时应尽量使用开放式提问,记录主诉时尽可能用患者自己描述的症状,不用诊断用语。主诉是用来确定中医的证,应尽量简洁。

主诉要素应简明扼要,与主症密切相关,从患者的角度表述发病原因。

3. 现病史 从此次发病开始至入院时疾病发生、发展的全过程。要求围绕主症,从辨证求因原则出发,记录疾病发生原因或诱因、发病时间、主症特点、病程进展、治疗经过以及必要的鉴别要点。

(1) 发病原因或诱因:尽可能了解疾病有无明显的病因和诱因。记录时应使用医学术语,根据起病特点恰当选用,要求言简意赅、确切表达。有的患者也可能把某个偶合情况当作病因或诱因,均应注意分析辨别。如果先后出现数个症状或体征,则应按顺序记录,如“情绪激动后出现心悸 3 个月,劳累后呼吸困难 2 周,下肢水肿 3 日”。

(2) 发病时间:记录症状开始出现的时间。

(3) 主症特点:① 具有同一性。即任何疾病的主症,必然与疾病主要矛盾相一致。② 具有运动性。即主症是运动变化的,它随着疾病主要矛盾的转化而改变。③ 具有变化性。即主症决定次要症状的出现,主症转变了,次要症状也随之转变。

例如:某女性患者患有风湿性关节炎 2 年,自觉双下肢疼痛 1 个月,遇寒加重,遇热痛减,关节屈伸不利,舌质淡、苔薄白、脉弦紧,中医辨证为寒痹,主症为双下肢冷痛 1 个月;3 个月后,该患者再次就诊,诉双下肢疼痛伴肿胀 2 周,痛有定处,肌肤麻木,苔白腻,脉濡缓,中医辨证为着痹,主症为双下肢疼痛伴肿胀 2 周。

(4) 治疗经过:本次就诊前已经接受过的诊断检查及其结果,中西医治疗所用药物的名称或是方药组成、剂量、给药途径、疗程及疗效,应记述清楚,以备制订诊断治疗方案时参考。

(5) 刻下:刻下是用来确定中医辨证的分型。主要记录患者目前的中医症状,包括舌苔脉象,可以参考《十问歌》帮助书写。中医症状能够反映中医证型。

4. 既往史 是指患者此次发病以前的健康状况及曾患疾病,应按时间顺序进行系统记录。

5. 系统回顾 在这个部分,医师会对患者身体所有的系统进行一个快速的检查,以期对诊断和治疗有所帮助。根据每个患者病情程度、临床表现和身体状况的不同,医师会对不同系统的检查有所偏重,有的系统可能很快地略过,有的系统可能需要花一定时间进行较为细致的检查(意味着会对患者询问更多的问题)。包括呼吸系统、循环系统、消化系统、生殖泌尿系统、造血系统、内分泌系统、肌肉骨骼系统、神经系统。

6. 个人史 包括生活情况,诞生地,居住环境,生活习惯,饮食嗜欲,运动情况,平素情志,烟酒药物情况。

7. 过敏史 对某些过敏原过敏的病史。过敏原包括:饮食性物质(如海鲜、果仁、草莓、香料、牛奶及酒精类饮品等)、空气传播性物质(如动物皮毛、尘螨、花粉、工业污染废料及霉菌等)、接触性物质(如化妆品、香水、指甲油及橡胶等)。

8. 婚姻史 应询问和记录婚姻状况(包括未婚、已婚、离异次数),结婚年龄,爱人健康状况。若配偶已死亡者,询问其死因和时间。

9. 月经史 记录初潮年龄、行经期、月经周期、末次月经时间(或绝经期)。

$$记录公式为:初潮年龄\frac{行经期天数}{月经周期天数}末次月经日期(或绝经年龄)$$

10. 产科史 记录孕育过孩子的妇女的妊娠次数、产次、分娩情况及存活数。记录公式为:$G*P*A*L*$,G 指的是怀孕次数 gestation,P 是指生产次数 production,A 是流产次数 abortion,L 是存活数 live。举例:$G_4P_2A_2L_1$ 具体指,这个妇女就是指怀孕 4 次,流产 2 次,生育 2 次,存活一个。

11. 家族史 主要记录患者父母、祖父母、兄弟、姐妹及子女的健康状况和发病情况,特别要注意中医认为与传染、遗传因素有关的病证。

12. 四诊合参 是中医诊断疾病的方法,包括望、闻、问、切,合称四诊。

(1)望:望诊是中医四诊中的第一部分。在望诊中,医师至少要观察患者四个方面的情况。首先,观察患者的整体情况,包括体型、行为举止、在就诊中的表现以及就诊中与医师之间的交流能力。其次,观察患者的面色(肤色)。再者,观察患者舌的情况,包括舌色、舌苔、舌的形状、舌下络脉和运动情况。最后,观察患者身体的分泌物和排泄物。以上四个方面都需要通过医师的观察,即望诊来实现。

(2)闻:包括听声音和嗅气味两个方面。听患者的说话声音、咳嗽、喘息以及嗅出患者的口臭、体臭等气味。

（3）问：在问诊中，询问患者一些很重要但是不容易获得的信息。在整个过程中，需要注意的是询问的问题是对于辨证有意义的。询问的问题包括以下内容（询问时需与中医《十问歌》相联系）：寒热、发汗、头痛、疼痛的性质和位置、大小便情况、饮食、睡眠、妇科情况以及个人情况（包括用药情况和心理、社会情况）。

（4）切：就是脉诊和触诊。脉诊就是切脉，掌握脉象。触诊，就是以手触按患者的体表病症部分，以助诊断。

13. 体格检查　是指医师运用自己的感官或借助于简单的评估工具对患者的身体进行细致的观察和系统的评估，以了解机体健康状况的最基本的一组评估方法。在进行体格检查时，切记顺序不能颠倒，以减少来回翻动患者，不给患者造成不便。同时对医师而言，依序检查也能防止有所遗漏。体格检查的评估方法包括：视诊、触诊、叩诊、听诊。具体内容如下。

（1）生命指征：体温、脉搏、呼吸、血压。

（2）一般情况：发育、营养、体型；神志：昏迷、嗜睡、是否清晰等；面容、表情；皮肤：颜色、皮疹、皮下出血、肝掌蜘蛛痣、皮下结节、水肿等；毛发。

（3）淋巴结。

（4）头面部

1）头颅：头颅大小、形态；头颅压痛、包块；头发。

2）眼：① 眉毛：观察有无脱落。② 眼睑：观察有无红肿、水肿，睑缘有无内翻或外翻，睫毛排列是否整齐以及生长方向，两侧眼睑是否对称，上睑提起及闭合功能是否正常。③ 结膜、巩膜：观察结膜的颜色，有无充血、水肿、乳头肥大、滤泡增生、瘢痕形成以及巩膜有无黄染。④ 角膜：观察透明度、有无白斑、云翳、溃疡、角膜软化和血管增生等。⑤ 瞳孔：观察瞳孔大小形状、直接间接对光反射、聚合反射。⑥ 眼球：外形、运动。⑦ 中医眼诊五轮检查：中医"五轮学说"是指将眼睛的不同部位分属五脏，即瞳仁属肾，称为水轮；黑睛属肝，称为风轮；两眦血络属心，称为血轮；白睛属肺，称为气轮；眼睑属脾，称为肉轮。通过观察五轮的形态、颜色、质地等变化，可以诊察相应脏腑的病变情况，对眼科临床和内科病症的诊断具有一定的意义。五轮与五脏、五行和现代解剖学位置的关系可见表6-1，中医眼诊五轮图可见图6-1。

表6-1　五轮与五脏、五行和现代解剖学位置的关系

五行	五脏	五轮	具体部位	现代解剖学位置
木	肝	风轮	黑睛	角膜
火	心	血轮	目内外眦	眦部皮肤、结膜、血管及泪阜、半月皱襞和泪点
土	脾	肉轮	眼睑	眼睑皮肤、皮下组织、肌肉、睑板和睑结膜
金	肺	气轮	白睛	球结膜、球筋膜和前部巩膜
水	肾	水轮	瞳神	狭义专指瞳孔；广义包括葡萄膜、视网膜、视神经以及房水、晶状体和玻璃状体等

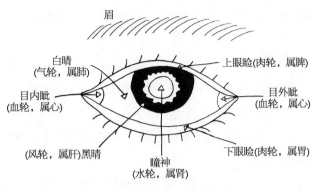

图 6-1　中医眼诊五轮图

3）耳：耳郭、外耳道、乳突。

4）中医耳诊：中医耳诊是一种诊断疾病、判断预后的诊断方法。耳是人体各脏腑组织器官的缩影，人体各脏器、各部位与耳部皆有集中反映点，脏腑组织有病必然反映于耳。因此，通过察耳可以窥知内脏之疾患。耳与脏腑组织相关图可见图 6-2。

5）鼻：鼻的外形、鼻翼翕动、鼻中隔、鼻窦以及鼻的通气状态。

6）口：口唇（观察色泽、有无疱疹、有无口角糜烂）、口腔黏膜、牙齿牙龈、舌、咽喉及扁桃体。

7）中医面诊：中医面诊是指透过面部反射区知道脏腑疾病与健康状况的诊断方法，从而能够快速大致掌握疾病的部位和特点。这是一种简单有效的发现疾病的方法，对于临床诊断具有非常重要的意义。中医面诊图可见图 6-3。

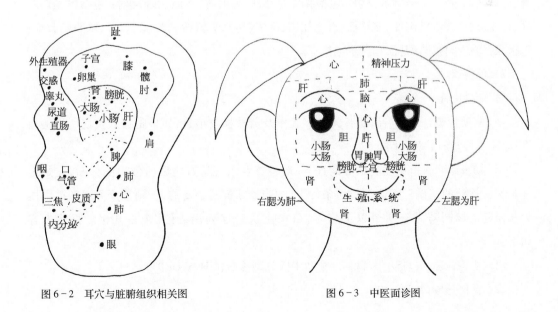

图 6-2　耳穴与脏腑组织相关图　　　　图 6-3　中医面诊图

（5）颈部　颈部外形、姿势运动、皮肤包块；颈部血管：颈静脉有无充盈、颈部动静脉搏动；甲状腺；气管。

（6）胸部

1）胸壁外形：① 胸壁：包括静脉、皮下气肿、胸壁压痛和肋间隙。② 乳房：观察两侧乳房的大小、对称性、外表、乳头状态及有无溢液等。

2）肺：观察呼吸类型、频率、深度、胸廓活动度、胸膜摩擦感，听诊肺部呼吸音、病理性呼吸音、啰音及胸膜摩擦音等。

3）心：心尖搏动：观察心尖搏动的位置、强度及范围、有无负性心尖搏动；震颤；心包摩擦感、心包摩擦音；心脏相对浊音界；心率、心音。

4）脊柱：观察脊柱弯曲度、活动度、压痛、叩击痛。

5）腹部：① 腹部外形、呼吸运动。② 腹壁：观察腹壁静脉、皮肤改变（包括皮疹、腹纹、手术瘢痕）、脐、疝；触诊腹壁紧张度、腹壁压痛、反跳痛（包括阑尾点、胆囊点）。③ 听诊腹部肠鸣音、振水音、血管杂音、移动性浊音、液波震颤。④ 腹内脏器：肝脏、胆囊、脾脏。⑤ 腹部包块。⑥ 腹壁反射。

6）四肢、神经系统：① 上肢：视诊上肢皮肤、关节、手指及指甲有无形态异常；上肢血管检查；观察上肢有无运动功能障碍或异常；上肢肌张力检查，注意两侧对比；上肢肌力检查，注意两侧对比；上肢生理反射：包括肱二头肌反射、肱三头肌反射、桡骨骨膜反射等；上肢病理反射：包括霍夫曼征等。② 下肢：视诊双下肢皮肤、下肢静脉、关节、踝部及趾甲；下肢血管检查；观察下肢有无运动功能障碍或异常；下肢肌张力检查，注意两侧对比；下肢肌力检查，注意两侧对比；下肢生理反射：包括膝反射、跟腱反射等；下肢病理反射：包括巴宾斯基征、查多克征、奥本海姆征、戈登征、贡达征、肌阵挛（包括髌阵挛和踝阵挛）等；脑膜刺激征：包括颈强直、布鲁津斯基征和凯尔尼格征。

7）舌苔、脉象。

8）专科检查。

14. 辅助检查　记录与诊断有关的实验室及器械检查结果，如果是在入院前所做的检查，应注明检查地点及日期。

15. 初步诊断　指在经过病史调查、一般检查及系统检查之后所做出的诊断，它是进一步实施诊疗的基础。无论在任何条件下，初步诊断都是必要的，否则诊疗方案和措施便无从谈起。诊断若是有两个以上病名，可按主次顺序列出，有几个写几个。具体内容如下：

（1）中医诊断：包括中医病名诊断和中医分型诊断（GB95，GB97）。

（2）西医诊断（ICD－10）。

16. 初步治疗 根据初步诊断制订的初步治疗方案,包括中医治疗和西医治疗。如Ⅱ级护理、普食/软食、理疗、静脉补液、针灸、中草药(内服或外用)、生活方式的调整、康复与锻炼。

17. 记录者签名 记录者必须签名。

(二)主治医师首次查房

主治医师查房每日 1 次,首次查房要求如下:病危者入院,当日要有上级医师(包括主治医师)查房;病重者入院后次日要有主治医师查房,一般患者入院后,主治医师首次查房不得超过 48 小时。常规查房要求如下:医嘱中病危者,上级查房(包括主治医师)每日 1 次;病重者,每日 1 次或者隔日 1 次。

主治医师查房,要求对所管患者分组进行系统查房。尤其对新入院、危重、诊断不明、治疗效果不好的患者进行重点检查与讨论,检查要做到望闻问切;听取医师和护士的反映;倾听患者的陈述,检查中医病历的书写情况并纠正其中错误的记录;了解病情变化并检查医嘱执行情况及治疗效果,调整中医治疗方案;决定出、转院问题。

病历书写中除了首次病程记录内容之外,还包括以下内容:西医鉴别诊断、中医类证鉴别、中医辨病辨证依据及分析。

(三)主任医师首次查房

每周查房 1 次。主任医师查房,要解决疑难病例:审查对新入院、危重患者诊断、治疗计划;决定特殊检查治疗,对患者要有望闻问切,检查并调整中医治疗方案(包括静脉滴注中药、口服中成药、中药饮片、针灸及其他中医治疗);抽查医嘱病历、监督中医病历质量、护理质量;听取医师、护士对诊疗护理的意见;进行必要的教学工作。

除以上内容外,主任医师查房病历中还应包括以下内容:治疗中应注意的问题、病情预后与转归、中医药及国内外学术进展。

举例:

患者某,男,50 岁。

主诉:气急喘促加重 3 日。

刻下症状:喘鸣,痰咳,胸闷,舌淡苔白滑,脉浮紧。

辨证分析(中医病因及病机):痰液在肺部的储存成为哮病发作的主要原因。水液的流通由肺、脾和肾完成。肺调节上焦水液通道,脾脏运输并转换中焦水液流通,肾脏支配下焦水液代谢。这三个器官中的阴阳不平衡导致水循环停滞,导致痰液生成和储存。因此,哮病的根本原因是痰的存在。这位患者因感受外邪而诱发哮病的急性发作。

鉴别诊断(辨病与辨证)：① 辨病——哮与喘："哮"和"喘"之间的区别是,哮的呼吸特点是哨笛的声音,而喘气是个人呼吸困难的感觉。哮以声音来命名。在喘气的时候,喉咙里的声音,就像青蛙的声音一样,称作哮。持续的加速呼吸不能停止称为喘。"喘必兼哮,哮未必兼喘"。他们都可以是哮喘的表现,与急性或慢性病程的侧重上不同。② 辨证——寒哮与热哮：寒哮,喉中如有水鸣声,痰色白。热哮,喉中喘鸣气粗,痰色黄。

治法：温肺散寒,化痰平喘。

内治方药：射干麻黄汤。

组成：射干9克,麻黄6克,干姜3克,细辛3克,半夏9克,厚朴9克,白前9克,杏仁9克。

加减：若痰涌喘息不得卧者,加葶苈子9克、白芥子9克;恶寒、发热、头痛者加荆芥9克、防风9克、桂枝6克;若鼻塞鼻痒,喷嚏频作加辛夷花6克。

外治法(穴位敷贴,灸法,针刺)：穴位敷贴。取大椎、天突穴,将白芥子15克、半夏15克,共研细末,用姜汁调成膏。将药膏分成2份敷贴在穴位上,用纱布覆盖,胶布固定。贴12小时后去药洗净,然后隔12小时再贴,共贴3次。

医嘱：调整饮食,注意保暖和休息,不能吸烟。

三、中医住院病历书写的要求

1. 中医住院病历书写要遵循相关法律法规 中医病历书写规范自2002年6月1日起实施,2010年进行了修订。中医病历记录首页应符合国家中医药管理局(SATCM)关于"中医医院医疗记录首页"(2001年第6条)的规定。特殊检查和特殊治疗应符合卫生部门对医疗机构实施条例(1994年)的有关规定。

2. 中医住院病历书写要体现中医特色,尽量使用中医术语 中医住院病历应体现中医特色,概括而言,即需要详细、准确、全面、有重点地,就四诊、八纲及具体辨证方法的需要,记录所搜集的资料,进一步加以综合分析,得出辨证(辨病)的结论,再系统地从理、法、方、药进行论治处理。

中医术语含有丰富的甚至是特异性的中医辨证信息,如口甜、口苦、自汗、盗汗、渴喜热饮等,但如果西医术语提供的信息对辨病更可靠、更科学,则可结合运用现代医学术语,以及体格检查、实验室检查结果的描述等。

总而言之,中医住院病历书写要把患者信息结合中医与西医的思路去分析,分别给出中医与西医的诊断,中医诊断要包括疾病和证型两部分,之后再给出中西医的治疗原则和具体治疗方案。诊断是整个中医住院病历中的重点。

3. **中医住院病历书写应注重客观事实** 客观、真实、重点突出、严禁虚构臆造，是病历书写的最基本要求。病历中所设项目，均应逐一认真填写，切忌任意涂改、填注。

4. **中医住院病历书写必须及时、规范、准确、完整** 病历书写的及时、规范、准确、完整，也是中医病历书写中的一个基本要求，与病历书写的客观、真实共同体现病历的客观性、科学性和法律性。

住院病历书写使用阿拉伯数字来记录日期和时间，时间使用 24 小时记录。一般中医住院病历由住院医师和在试用期的医师来书写，之后由上级医师进行修改和签字。一般使用蓝黑水笔进行书写，其他颜色的水笔或是圆珠笔是不能进行病历书写的。

入院记录 24 小时内完成，首次病程记录 8 小时内完成，抢救记录及时完成，未能及时完成的必须在 6 小时内补记。手术记录应在 24 小时内完成，术后病程记录应在术后即时完成。非手术患者诊疗知情记录在入院后 72 小时内完成，出院或死亡记录在患者出院或死亡后 24 小时内完成。法定传染病按规定及时报告并在病程记录中及时记录。病程记录中对危重患者根据病情随时记录，至少每日记录 1 次，病情稳定的患者至少 3 日 1 次，病情稳定的慢性病患者至少 5 日记录 1 次。新患者入院后及一般手术后 3 日内每日进行病程记录（不同地区可能有不同要求）。

5. **中医住院病历书写必须充分尊重患者知情权并在病历中体现** 知情选择作为患者的权利，已为医患双方所认同，在中医医院病历书写中，也应充分考虑这一点。

告知书、委托书、授权书、诊疗知情同意书、手术麻醉知情同意书等均应严格遵守有关规定，认真予以执行。知情告知既忌过分夸大病情引起患者恐慌，又必须避免带着一种主观意向或者凭着一种良好愿望去吸引患者、引导患者。另外如患者的特殊检查、特殊治疗、特殊用药、输血等均应充分告知并征得同意。此外，必须注意告知书的签字日期及签字人身份，患者能自己签署的必须由患者本人签署。特殊情况者必须按有关规定由患者的法定代理人、近亲属或关系人签署。

四、一般注意事项

1. 进行体格检查时的注意事项

（1）体格检查必须认真、仔细，按部位和系统顺序进行，重要的是检查顺序不能颠倒，以减少来回翻动患者，不给患者造成不便，同时对医师而言，依序检查也不至于有所遗漏。

（2）既有所侧重，又不遗漏阳性体征。

（3）对患者态度要和蔼、严肃，集中思想，手法轻柔，注意患者反应，冷天要注意保暖。

（4）对危急患者可先重点检查，及时进行抢救处理，待病情稳定后再做详细检查；不要过多搬动，以免加重病情。

2. 书写中医住院病历时的注意事项

（1）在患者住院期间，其完整的住院病历应该随时都可供使用。

（2）住院病历上的每一页都应包含患者的姓名、住院号和所住病房位置。

（3）住院病历的书写应该有一个统一的标准和格式。

（4）住院病历的书写应该反映患者护理治疗过程的连续性，并且应该按照时间顺序来查看。

（5）在入院、交接和出院时记录或沟通的病历应采用标准化的形式进行记录书写。

（6）住院病历的每次书写都应该记录下日期、时间（采取 24 小时制），而且书写的内容应能被辨认，且记录者需要签名。除了手写草书签名外，记录者还应进行可辨识的正规签名。关于病历的删除和修改都应该记录日期、时间并签名。

（7）病历记录应该尽快在患者收治入院后、查房后或是相关工作人员下班前完成。如果有延迟，则应记录下延迟的时间和此次延迟记录的发生。

（8）每一次病历记录都应该经过做此次医嘱的本医疗机构注册的医务人员审阅。

（9）每一次负责患者护理的护理人员的变动都应记录下姓名、日期和时间。

（10）每当医师看过患者，都应该在病历上进行记录。当在医院的病历记录中有超过 4 日的急性医疗治疗或超过 7 日的长期连续性治疗没有记录时，要在新的病历中记录原因。

（11）出院记录/出院单应该在患者入院时便开始记录。

（12）必须在病历记录中清楚地记录患者拒绝治疗、同意治疗、心肺复苏的决定。在患者不是决定者的情况下，做决定的人应该是由患者确认的，如律师。

五、中医住院病历的作用

中医住院病历既是临床实践工作的总结，又是探索疾病规律及处理医疗纠纷的法律依据。为此，医护人员在书写中医住院病历时一定要实事求是、严肃认真、科学严谨、一丝不苟。中医住院病历对医疗、教学、科研、医院管理、预防疾病和法律都有重要的作用。

1. 医疗　中医住院病历既是确定诊断、进行治疗、落实预防措施的资料，又是医务人员诊治疾病水平评估的依据，也是患者再次患病时诊断与治疗的重要参考资料。通过临床病历回顾，可以从中汲取经验、教训，改进工作，提高医疗质量。

2. 教学　中医住院病历是教学的宝贵资料，是最生动的教材。通过中医住院病历的书写与阅读，可以使医务人员所学的医学理论和医疗实践密切结合起来，巩固所学知识，开阔视野，培养医务人员和医学生的逻辑思维能力，形成严谨的医疗作风。

3. 科研　中医住院病历是临床研究的主要素材。通过临床病历总结分析，寻求疾病发生、发展、治疗转归的客观规律及内在联系,研究临床治疗、预防措施与疾病、康复的关系,发现筛选新的医疗技术和药物,推动医学不断发展。

4. 医院管理 大量的中医住院病历资料分析可以客观地反映医院工作状况、技术素质、医疗质量、管理措施、医德医风等医院管理水平。因此,检查病历、分析病历,从中发现问题、解决问题,是了解医院工作状态、提高医疗质量的重要手段之一,也是提高医院管理水平的重要措施。

5. 预防疾病 通过对病历的分类统计和分析,可以了解临床各种常见病、多发病的发生与发展情况,为控制和落实预防措施、贯彻预防为主的方针提供依据。

6. 法律 中医住院病历是处理医疗事故、医疗纠纷的法律依据。因此,中医住院病历是有效地保护患者和医务人员合法权益的重要文件。

六、阅读材料

(1) 朱文,朱杰.统一中西医病历格式——谈中医病历管理存在的问题与对策[J].现代医院,2014,14(10):96.

(2) 病历书写编委会.病历书写基本规范(2010 版)[S].北京:人民卫生出版社,2010.

七、课后习题

22 岁的女性。

主诉:心悸复发 1 个月。

病史:1 个月前,无明显诱因下,出现心悸,心悸不甚,无胸痛,无晕厥,呼吸急促,无下肢水肿,无上臂震颤,无发热,胃纳可。伴盗汗,颧红,口渴欲饮,尿短赤,大便秘结,舌红少津,脉细数。无传染病史,对海鲜过敏。未婚,月经正常。

由标准化患者(SP 患者)问诊后,请完成一份中医住院病历。

参考文献

[1] 医疗保险和医疗补助服务中心.个人健康记录[EB/OL].[2012 – 04 – 14].https://www.cms.gov/
 Medicare/E-Health/PerHealthRecords.

Chapter Six

TCM Inpatient Record Writing

This chapter is divided into following parts: definition, the structure of inpatient record writing, the regulations and guidelines of inpatient record writing, general tips, function of inpatient record writing, suggesting reading after class and homework.

1. Definition

The term medical record is used somewhat interchangeably to describe the systematic documentation of a single patient's medical history and care across time within one particular health care provider's jurisdiction. The medical record is the firsthand information of health care, medical education and scientific research. Meanwhile, the medical record provides not only important basis for health care quality evaluation and hospital management decision, but also original evidence for medical insurance and medical dispute and malpractice. A good medical record is also a key indicator to measure doctor's professional skill. Therefore, medical record writing is of significant importance.

The medical record includes outpatient record and inpatient record. Inpatient record writing is a basic technique for each doctor. Through the process of inpatient record writing, doctor can enhance the ability of collecting medical history and performing physical examination, improve the communication with patients, train the thinking ability of clinical diagnosis and differential diagnosis, and cultivate the ability to adjust the treatment according to the disease condition. Inpatient record writing is a basic technique for each doctor, including a series of documents.

TCM possesses its own theoretical system and characteristics of syndrome differentiation. The benchmark of TCM is "Zheng", which means doctors should observe internal state of disease and pathogenesis through external Zheng symptoms, thus analyzing the cause, location, nature and mechanism of the disease on the basis of its development condition. It requires not only the detailed disease record of outbreak, manifestation, development and evolvement, but also the whole practice record of diagnosis, treatment and therapeutic effect. Therefore, TCM inpatient record has unique features, besides medical history collection and physical examination of WM, the patients' information collecting by TCM four diagnostic methods should also be recorded in detail, and analyzed inductively which embodies the thinking process of syndrome differentiation and treatment, thereby confirming TCM disease and syndrome diagnosis and formulating TCM treatment plan. In other words, an intact and outstanding TCM inpatient record requires not only the detailed disease record of outbreak, manifestation, development and evolvement, but also the whole practice record of diagnosis, treatment and therapeutic effect.

Main records for inpatients include: Patient note/Admission note (24 hrs), initial progress note (8 hrs), record of attending round (48 hrs), record of chief round, progress note.

2. The Structure of Inpatient Record Writing

Most important is preciseness, in time, integrity, consistency.

Here is an intact content of what is involved in TCM inpatient record.

2.1 Initial progress note (8 hrs)

2.1.1　General information: Including patient's name, age, gender, race, nationality, address, occupation, marital status, date of admission, date of record, complainer of history insurance information and telephone contact details.

2.1.2　Chief complaint: Chief complaint is the main reason the patient is seeking care for including the obvious symptom and/or sign, nature of the disease and duration. Asking open ended questions will help gain information about the chief complaint. When writing down the chief complaint, try to use patients' own description, not diagnostic terms. Chief complaint should be as brief as possible. Chief complaint is used to determine the "Zheng" of TCM.

Chief complaint should be concise, directly link to main condition, address the reason for encounter from patient's aspect.

2.1.3　Present history: Present history is the whole process from the onset to the development of disease. Doctor should follow the principle that centering on chief complaint to make diagnosis and treatment. Present history includes cause and inducement of disease, time since onset, characteristics of main symptoms, progress, previous treatment and present signs and/or symptoms and necessary differentiation (WM+TCM).

2.1.3.1　Cause and inducement of disease: Try best to know if patient has obvious cause and inducement of disease. According to the clinical characters, use proper medical terms in the record to express correctly and briefly. Sometimes patient may regard accidental condition as cause or inducement of disease, doctor should distinguish the truth from false. When there are several symptoms and signs, doctor should record them in order. For example, palpitation after being emotional for 3 months, dyspnea after tired for 2 weeks, edema of lower extremities for 3 days.

2.1.3.2　Time since onset: record the time since symptoms and signs appear.

2.1.3.3　Characteristics of main symptoms

2.1.3.3.1　Identity: The main symptoms should correspond with the main conflicts of diseases.

2.1.3.3.2　Mutability: The main symptoms are constantly changing with the main conflicts of diseases.

2.1.3.3.3　Variability: The main symptoms determine the secondary symptoms. If the main symptoms change, the secondary symptoms change with them.

For example, a female patient has been diagnosed with rheumatoid arthritis for 2 years. Her lower extremities were painful for 1 month, the pain aggravated with cold weather while alleviated with warm weather, the joints were inhibited in bending and stretching, pale tongue had thin white coating and the pulse was tight and wiry.

TCM diagnosis was cold Bi syndrome and main symptom was cold pain in lower extremities for 1 month. After 3 months, she came to the clinic again with painful and swollen lower extremities for 2 weeks. The pain was fixed, and the skin was numb. The tongue was white with a white greasy coating and the pulse was soggy and moderate. This time TCM diagnosis was damp Bi syndrome and main symptoms were painful and swollen lower extremities for 2 weeks.

2.1.3.4　Previous treatment: Including previous diagnostic test result and treatment before hospitalization. Western medical drug names and/or TCM prescription including its composition, dosage, administration route, course of treatment and curative effect should be clearly recorded for making further treatment plan use.

2.1.3.5　Present symptoms: Present symptoms are used to diagnose the TCM pattern. Present symptoms mainly record the current TCM symptoms including tongue, tongue coating and pulse. Present symptoms record writing can refer to TCM *Ten Question Songs*. TCM symptoms can reflect TCM pattern.

2.1.4   Previous history: Previous history means patient's premorbid state of health and illness which should be recorded systematically according to the time order.

2.1.5   Review of systems: In this section, doctor takes a quick glance at all of the system of the body to determine if more follow up is needed. Depending on the patients and their health, for some systems the doctor may only take a few seconds to ask about, whereas other systems may have a few minutes or more devoted to them if a patient indicates a problem or issue (more follow up questions can be done to get more information). Systems include respiratory system、 circulatory system、 alimentary system、 genitourinary system、 hematopoietic system、 endocrine system、 skeletal and muscle system、 neural system.

Exercise 1: 30 years old male, recurrent diarrhea for 3 months.

Exercise 2: 50 years old female, menstruation stopped for 3 months.

Exercise 3: 33 years old female, joint pain for 8 months.

2.1.6   Personal history: Personal history includes patient's life condition, place of born, living environment, living habit, diet, current activities of daily life, personal emotion, current travel history, alcohol, drug and smoking.

2.1.7   Allergy history: Medical history about some allergens, which include eating substances such as seafood, nuts, strawberry, spice, milk and alcoholic beverages, airborne substances such as animal fur, dust mite, pollen, industrial waste and mold, contact substances such as cosmetics, perfume, nail polish and latex.

2.1.8   Marital history: Ask and record patient's marital status including spinsterhood/married/divorced, marriage time, and spouse health status. If patient has been bereft of his/her spouse, doctor should ask and record his/her cause of death and death time.

2.1.9   Menstrual history: (Female only) record age of menarche, menstrual period, menstrual cycle and the last menstrual period or menopause. The formula can be written as follows:

$$\text{age of menarche} \ \frac{\text{menstrual period(days)}}{\text{menstrual cycle(days)}} \ \text{the last menstrual period or menopause age}$$

2.1.10   Obstetrical history: (Female only) record number of pregnancies, number of labors, delivery conditions and survival number. The formula can be written as follows: $G*P*A*L*$. G means gestation, P means production, A means abortion or miscarriage, and L means Live number. For example, $G_4P_2A_2L_1$ means the female patient had 4 gestations, 2 productions, 2 abortions and one to live (Abortions usually refer to terminations; For natural early pregnancy loss present terminology is miscarriages).

2.1.11 Family history: Mainly record the health status and disease situation of patient's parents, grandparents, brothers, sisters and offspring, especially noting disease which is related to contagious and genetic factors in TCM theory.

2.1.12 TCM four diagnostic methods: Including inspection, auscultation and olfaction, inquiry and pulse-taking.

2.1.12.1 Inspection: The first stage of TCM four diagnostic methods is inspection. In inspection examination, the doctor attends to at least four characteristics that are visible to the eye. The first is general appearance, including the patient's physical shape, the patient's manner, the way he or she behaves during the clinical encounter, and the quality of the patient-doctor interaction. The second is facial color (complexion). The third characteristic is the tongue, including the material of the tongue itself (color), the coating of the tongue, its shape and the veins and movement. The fourth is the bodily secretions and excretions. These characteristics are presented in the order of observation by the doctor.

2.1.12.2 Auscultation and olfaction: Auscultation includes listening to the speak voice and internal sound made by patient's body such as cough and wheezing. Olfaction includes distinguish the internal scents made by patient's body such as ozostomia and body odor.

2.1.12.3 Inquiry: In this part, doctor asks questions to discover important but not readily apparent information. Of course, many questions may be asked, but only those that are most common and that essential for doctors to learn pattern perception are discussed here. These cover the following topics (which are related to TCM ten question song): sensations of cold or hot; perspiration; headaches and dizziness; quality and location of pain; urination and stool; thirst; appetite and tastes; sleep; gynecological concerns; and personal background (including medical and psychosocial history).

2.1.12.4 Pulse: Taking and population: Part of diagnostic process involves taking pulse and touching different part of the body to help diagnose.

2.1.13 Physical examination: Physical examination is the most basic evaluation method understanding patient's health condition that doctor uses their own sense organ or simple evaluation tool to observe and assess patient's body. Physical examination should be taken in order which brings two benefits which can reduce the times of position change for patient and can also prevent health provider from missing some part of examination. The evaluation methods include inspection, palpation, percussion and auscultation.

2.1.13.1 Vital signs: body temperature (T), respiration rate (RR), pulse rate (PR), and blood pressure (BP).

2.1.13.2   General condition

2.1.13.2.1   Development situation, nutrition, body type.

2.1.13.2.2   Consciousness: Coma/lethargy/clear mind or not.

2.1.13.2.3   Facial features and expression.

2.1.13.2.4   Skin: Color, rash, subcutaneous hemorrhage, liver palms, spider angioma, subcutaneous nodules, edema, etc.

2.1.13.2.5   Hair.

2.1.13.2.6   Lymph gland.

2.1.13.3   Head and face region

2.1.13.3.1   Head: Size and shape, tenderness and mass, hair.

2.1.13.3.2   Eye: Eyebrow: observe if it has shed or not.

Eyelid: observe if it is red, swollen, puffy, introversive or extravertive. Observe the eyelash is lined or not. Look at the eyelid in both sides, comparing for symmetry. Ask patient to move his/her upper eyelid to observe its function.

Conjunctiva and sclera: observe the color of conjunctiva. Whether the conjunctiva is congestive, dropsically or not. Whether there is papillary hypertrophy, follicular hyperplasia, scar formation or not. Whether sclera is stained yellow or not.

Cornea: observe its transparency. Whether there is vitiligo, nebula, ulceration, keratomalacia, vascular proliferation or not.

Pupil: observe its size and shape, direct and indirect light reflex, convergence reflex. Eyeball: observe its shape and movement.

TCM five orbiculi examination: TCM five orbiculi theory means different parts of eyes represent the five internal organs. Pupil belongs to kidney which is called water orbiculi. Cornea belongs to liver which is called wind orbiculi. Canthus belongs to heart which is called blood orbiculi. Eye white belongs to lung which is called Qi orbiculi. Eyelid belongs to spleen which is called flesh orbiculi. Through observing the shape, color and texture of five orbiculi, health providers can know the disease development of the five internal organs, which is of much importance to the diagnosis of ophthalmology and internal medical diseases. The relationship among TCM five orbiculi, five internal organs, five elements and modern anatomy location can be seen in Table 6 - 1. The picture of TCM five orbiculi can be seen in Figure 6 - 1.

Table 6－1 **The relationship among TCM five orbiculi, five internal organs,**
five elements and modern anatomy location

Five elements	Five internal organs	TCM five orbiculi	TCM location	Modern anatomy location
Wood	Liver	Wind orbiculi	Cornea	Cornea
Fire	Heart	Blood orbiculi	Canthus	The skin, conjunctiva, blood vessel of canthus and carunculae lacrimalis, plica semilunaris and dacryon
Earth	Spleen	Flesh orbiculi	Eyelid	The skin, subcutaneous tissue and muscle of eyelid and tarsus and palpebral conjunctiva
Metal	Lung	Qi orbiculi	Eye white	Bulbar conjunctiva, tenon's capsule and anterior scleritis
Water	Kidney	Water orbiculi	Pupil	Narrow sense means pupil and broad sense includes uvea, retina, optic nerve, aqueous fluid, lens and vitreous bod

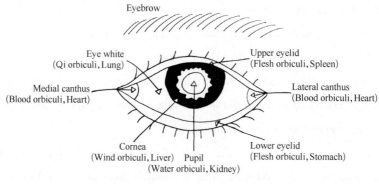

Figure 6－1　The picture of TCM five orbiculi

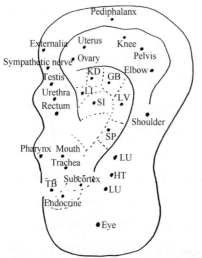

LV=Liver, HT=Heart, LU=Lung, SP=Spleen, KD–Kidney, GB=Gallbladder, SI=Small intestine, LI=Large intestine, TB=Triple burner

Figure 6－2　The relationship between ear and internal organs

2.1.13.3.3　Ear: Observe auricle, external auditory canal and mastoid process

TCM ear diagnosis: TCM ear diagnosis is a method to diagnose disease and judge prognosis. In TCM, ear can reflect internal organs in human body. Different organs of body has its own point in ear. Therefore, doctor can inspect ear to know the disease of internal organ. The relationship between ear and internal organs can be seen in Figure 6－2.

2.1.13.3.4　Nose: Observe its shape, nasal flaring, ventilation status of nasal septum, nasal sinus and nose.

2.1.13.3.5　Mouth：Lips（observe colour and lustre，with or without herpes and perleche）, mucous membrane, teeth, gums, tongue, throat and tonsil.

2.1.13.3.6　TCM face diagnosis：TCM face diagnosis is a diagnostic method. Doctor can know the location and characteristics of diseased organ and health status through facial reflecting region. It is a simple and effective method to find disease, and also very meaningful in diagnosing clinical disease. The picture of TCM face diagnosis can be seen in Figure 6 – 3.

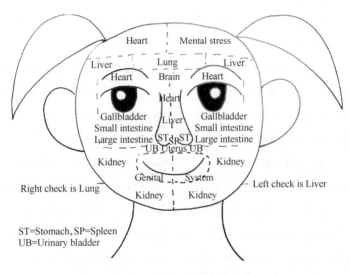

Figure 6 – 3　The picture of TCM face diagnosis

2.1.13.4　Neck region：a. Shape, posture, movement and mass. b. Blood vessel：whether there is jugular vein distention, carotid pulsation, jugular vein pulsation or not. c. Thyroid. d. Trachea.

2.1.13.5　Thorax region

2.1.13.5.1　Shape：a. Thoracic wall：includes vein, subcutaneous emphysema, tenderness and intercostal space. b. Breast：observe size, symmetry, appearance and nipple. Whether nipple has discharge or not.

2.1.13.5.2　Lung：observe breath type, respiratory rate, respiratory depth, thoracic activity and sense of pleural friction. Listen to the chest to see whether there is lung breath sounds, abnormal breath sounds and pleural friction sounds.

2.1.13.5.3　Heart：a. Apical impulse：observe its location, strength and range. Whether there is negative apical impulse. b. Tremor. c. Sensation and sounds of pericardia frication.

d. Relative cardiac dullness. e. Heart rate and heart sounds.

2.1.13.6   Spine: observe curvature, activity, tenderness and percussion pain.

2.1.13.7   Abdomen region: a. Abdominal shape and respiratory movement. b. Abdominal wall: observe abdominal wall vein, the skin change (including rash, abdominal striate and surgical scar), navel and hernia. Palpate the abdominal wall to feel the rigidity, tenderness, rebound tenderness (including McBurney's point and gallbladder point). c. Listen to the bowel sounds, succession splash sounds, vascular murmur, shifting dullness and fluid thrill. d. Intra-abdominal organs: liver, gallbladder and spleen. e. Abdominal mass. f. Abdominal reflex.

2.1.13.8   Extremities and Nervous System

2.1.13.8.1   Upper extremities. a. Observe the skin, joint, finger and nail. b. Blood vessel. c. Motor function. d. Muscle tone: compare in both sides. e. Muscle strength: compare in both sides. f. Physiological reflex: includes biceps reflex, triceps reflex and radio periosteal reflex, etc. g. Pathological reflex: includes Hoffmann sign, etc.

2.1.13.8.2   Lower extremities. a. Observe the skin, vein, joint, ankle and toenail. b. Blood vessel. c. Motor function. d. Muscle tone: compare in both sides. e. Muscle strength: compare in both sides. f. Physiological reflex: includes knee reflex and ankle reflex, etc. g. Pathological reflex: includes Babinski sign, Chaddock sign, Oppenheim sign, Gordon sign, Gonda sign, myoclonus (patellar clonus and ankle clonus), etc. h. Meningeal irritation sign: includes cervical rigidity, Brudzinski sign and Kernig sign.

2.1.13.9   Tongue and Pulse.

2.1.13.10   Specialty examination.

2.1.14   Auxiliary examination: Record every laboratory and instrumental examination result related to the diagnosis. If the patient has a prehospital examination, the examination place and date should be noted.

2.1.15   Primary diagnosis: primary diagnosis means the diagnosis is made after disease history collecting, general and systematic examination. It is the base of further treatment. Under any condition, it is necessary to make a primary diagnosis; otherwise, there is no treatment plan. If there are two or more than two primary diagnoses, they should be recorded in order of priority.

2.1.15.1   TCM diagnosis: includes TCM disease and pattern (GB95, GB97).

2.1.15.2   Western Medicine diagnosis (ICD − 10)

2.1.16   Primary treatment plan: Primary treatment plan is made according to the primary diagnosis which includes TCM and WM treatment. For example, level 2 nursing, general diet/

soft food, physical therapy, intravenous drips or injection, acupuncture & moxibustion, herbal therapy (oral or external), adjustment of lifestyle, rehabilitation and exercise.

2.1.17   Signature — doctor must sign his or her name.

2.2   Record of attending round (48 hrs)   Ward rounds should be made once a day. The first ward rounds are required as follows: for critical ill patients, attending physicians are required to make ward rounds on the admission day. For the patients with severe diseases, attending physicians should make ward rounds the next day after admission. For general patients, the first ward rounds by the attending physician should not exceed 48 hours after admission. Routine ward rounds are required as follows: for the critically ill patients, the ward rounds should be made once a day. For the patients with severe diseases, once a day or every other day.

The attending physician are required to make systematic rounds in groups. Especially for the new admission patients, the patients with critical, unclear diagnosis and the patients with less treatment effect, attending physicians should focus on the examination and discussion including TCM four diagnosis methods. During ward rounds, attending physician should hear from residents and nurses, listen to the patients, check the writing of TCM medical records and correct the wrong records, check the implementation of the doctor's advice and treatment effect, adjust to the treatment plan of TCM and decide discharge and transfer.

Besides the above contents in initial progress note, record of attending round should also include:

2.2.1   Differential diagnosis of WM.

2.2.2   Syndrome differentiation of TCM.

2.2.3   Dialectical basis and analysis of disease differentiation of TCM.

2.3   Record of chief round   Ward rounds should be made once a week. Chief rounds are required to solve difficult cases, review the diagnosis and treatment plan, determine the special examination and treatment, apply TCM four diagnosis methods, check and adjust TCM treatment including Chinese patent medicine, Chinese herbal decoction, acupuncture and other TCM treatments. Also, the chief physician should randomly inspect the records in order to supervise the quality of TCM inpatient records. The Chief physician should listen to the other doctors' and nurses' suggestions. Teaching jobs should be done, as necessary.

In addition, record of chief round should also include: a. Key problems in treatment. b. Prognosis and outcome of the disease. c. Academic process of TCM and medical science at home and abroad.

For example:

Name: XX; Gender: male; Age: 50y.

Chief compliant: Wheezing aggravated for 3 days.

Present symptoms: wheezing, cough with sputum and chest tightness, pale tongue; white slippery tongue coating, floating tense pulse.

Analysis of the disease in etiology and pathology: For this patient, the storage of phlegm in the Lung becomes the main cause for recurrent asthma attacks. Lung, Spleen, and Kidney control the passage of water. Lung regulates the water passages in the upper Jiao, the Spleen transports and transforms water in the middle Jiao, and Kidney dominates water metabolism in the lower Jiao. Imbalance of Yin and Yang in any of these three organs may lead to stagnation of the water circulation, which then contributes to the production and storage of phlegm in the Lung. The fundamental cause of asthma is the presence of phlegm.

Because of these, the patient is suffered from exogenous pathogenic agent, which induces the acute onset of wheezing syndrome.

Differentiation of disease and syndrome: a. Differentiation between disease: wheezing and panting. Wheezing is characterized by a whistling sound, while panting is when individuals have difficulty breathing. Wheezing is named for the sound, panting is named for the breath. During periods of panting, a sound in the throat, like the sound of a frog, is called wheezing. Persistent accelerated breathing with inability to stop is called panting. Wheezing necessarily occurs combined with panting, but panting can occur alone. Both can be manifestations of asthma and related to acute or chronic disease. b. Differentiation of syndrome: cold and heat. Cold-wheezing: frog-croak-like gurgling in the throat with white clear phlegm. Hot-wheezing: coarse and gurgling wheeze in the throat with sticky yellow phlegm.

Therapeutic methods: to warm the lung, dispel cold, resolve phlegm, and relieve wheezing.

Prescription:

Internal therapy: Shegan Mahuang Tang.

Shegan 9 g, Mahuang 6 g, Ganjiang 3 g, Xixin 3 g, Banxia 9 g, Baiqian 9 g, Xingren 9 g.

Modification: a. For severe dyspnea with abundant sputum and inability to lie flat, add Tinglizi 9 g and Baijiezi 9 g. b. For aversion to cold, fever and headache, add Jingjie 9 g, Fangfeng 9 g, Guizhi 6 g. c. For itching nose, nasal obstruction and frequent sneezing, add Xinyihua 6 g.

External therapy: Baijiezi 15 g, Banxia 15 g. Pulverize the drugs and mix the powder with ginger juice, prepare it into paste, and divide it into 2 portions. Apply the paste on Dazhui, Tiantu, cover the past with gauze and fix with adhesive plaster for 12 hours. Once daily, with 3 times as a treatment course.

Advice: light flavored, be careful of your diet (well-cooked diet), keep warm and rest, do not smoke.

3. The Regulations and Guidelines of Inpatient Record Writing

3. 1 Inpatient record writing should obey the related laws and regulations The basic norms of TCM record writing have been implemented since July 1, 2002, and revised in 2010. TCM record home page should conform to the state administration of traditional Chinese medicine (SATCM) about "the Chinese medicine hospital medical record home page" ([2001] no. 6). Special examination and special treatment should be in accordance with "the regulations of medical institution implementation rules" the relevant provisions of the health ministry (1994).

3. 2 Inpatient record should be written on (complying with) the principle of TCM characteristics and use TCM terms as far as possible Inpatient record should be written on the principle of TCM characteristics. In general, firstly, doctors use TCM four diagnostic methods, eight-principle syndrome differentiation and concrete diagnostic methods to record collecting data minutely, accurately, roundly and selectively. Secondly, collected data should be analyzed comprehensively to make a diagnosis. Last, doctor makes a treatment plan on the base of principle-method-recipe-medicines.

TCM terms possess abundant and specific TCM diagnostic information, such as sweet taste, bitter taste, spontaneous sweating, night sweating, thirst and desire for hot drinks, thirst but no desire to drink, etc. But if WM terms are more reliable and more scientific to diagnose the disease, doctor should combine TCM, WM terms and results of physical examination and laboratory examination.

That is to say, in TCM inpatient record writing, clinical manifestation data need to be organized and analyzed in both WM and TCM way. WM diagnosis and TCM diagnosis (disease + pattern) should be written. Then WM and TCM treatment principle and therapy should be given. All in all, diagnosis is of great concern in TCM inpatient recording writing.

3. 3　Inpatient record writing should pay attention to objective reality　The most basic requirement of inpatient record writing is following the principles of objectivity, reality, emphasis and no fiction or fabrication. Every item in the record should be written truly one by one without any amendment.

3. 4　Inpatient record writing should be in time, formal, accurate and intact　The other basic requirement of inpatient record writing is following the principles of timeliness, formalization, accuracy and integrity. Combined with objectivity and reality, inpatient record shows reasonability and legality.

Inpatient record writing uses Arabic numerals to write the date and time, using 24-hour record time. The records are written by interns, medical and staffs in probation period. And the records should be reviewed and modified and signed by the medical personnel qualified. Use blue or black ink pen to write, other color pen or ball — pen is forbidden and invalid.

Resident admit note should be completed within 24 hours, the first progress note within 8 hours and first-aid note immediately. If first-aid note can't be done immediately, it should be completed within 6 hours. Operation note should be completed within 24 hours, post operation progress note immediately, informed treatment record of non-surgical inpatient 72 hours after admission to hospital, discharge record 24 hours after discharge, death note 24 hours after death. Statutory infectious disease should be recorded by rule in progress note timely. To critical patient, according to their disease condition, progress note should be recorded at least once per day. For common patients, once every three days. The progress note of new admission patient and common operation patient should be recorded everyday within 3 days. Different countries may have different requirements.

3. 5　Inpatient record writing should fully respect patient's right and the right should be embodied in the record　Informed choice, as patient's right, has been acknowledged by both sides of health care. In inpatient record writing, doctors should fully take it into consideration.

Notification, letter of authorization and information consent form should be recorded according to relevant provisions. Informed consent can neither exaggerate the disease nor guide the patients with doctor's subjective intention. Other procedures such as special examination, special treatment, special medications and blood transfusion should all be fully informed of to gain patient's agreement. Furthermore, the date of signature and the identity of signatory should be noted. In principle, patients should sign the informed letter by themselves, but if the patients cannot sign the letter by themselves, the letter could be signed by the legal representative, immediate relatives or related privy of the patients.

4. General Tips

4. 1 Tips in performing physical examination

4. 1.1 Doctor must adhere to serious attitude to perform physical examination according to the site and system. Physical examination should be taken in order which brings two benefits. One is, for patient, to reduce the times of position change and the other is to prevent doctor from missing some part of examination.

4. 1.2 Doctors should make a distinction between the relatively important examinations and the lesser one without missing any positive sign.

4. 1.3 Doctors should show kind manners to the patients and pay attention to patient's reaction. Be sure to keep warm in winter.

4. 1.4 Doctors can preferentially perform main examination to critical patients. When patients are in a stable condition, doctors can do the rest. Don't move the critical patients too many times in case aggravating the disease.

4. 2 Tips in writing inpatient record

4.2.1 The patient's complete medical record should be available at all times during their stay in hospital.

4.2.2 Every page in the medical record should include the patient's name, identification number (NHS number) and location in the hospital.

4.2.3 The contents of the medical record should have a standardized structure and layout.

4.2.4 Documentation within the medical record should reflect the consecutiveness of patient care and should be viewable in chronological order.

4.2.5 Data recorded or communicated on admission, handover and discharge should be recorded using a standardized format.

4.2.6 Every entry in the medical record should be dated, timed (24-hour clock), legible and signed by the person making the entry. The name and designation of the person making the entry should be legibly printed besides their signature. Deletions and alterations should be countersigned, dated and timed.

4.2.7 Entries to the medical record should be made as soon as possible after the event is documented (e.g. change in clinical state, ward round, investigation) or before the relevant staff member goes off duty. If there is a delay, the time of the event and the delay should be recorded.

4.2.8　Every entry in medical record should be identified by the most senior healthcare professional person (who is responsible for decision making).

4.2.9　On each occasion the consultant who is responsible for the patient's care changes, the name of the new responsible consultant and the date and time of the agreed transfer of care, should be recorded.

4.2.10　An entry should be made in the medical record whenever a patient is seen by a doctor. When there is no entry in the hospital record for more than four days for acute medical care or seven days for long-stay continuing care, the next entry should explain why.

4.2.11　The discharge record/discharge summary should be commenced at the time a patient is admitted to hospital.

4.2.12　Advanced decisions to refuse treatment, consent and cardio-pulmonary resuscitation decisions must be clearly recorded in the medical record. In circumstances where the patient is not the decision maker, that person should be identified, e.g., attorney.

5. Function of Inpatient Record Writing

TCM inpatient record writing is not only the summary of clinical practice, but also legal basis in exploring disease rules and dealing with medical disputes. For this reason, when writing inpatient record, doctors must seek truth from facts and hold the scientific and rigorous attitude. TCM inpatient record plays a significant role in health care, medical teaching, scientific research, hospital management, disease prevention and legislation.

5.1　Health care　TCM inpatient record has three identities: the data for diagnosing, treating and preventing the disease, the reference for evaluating doctors' diagnostic and therapeutic level, and the reference materials for further diagnose and treatment. Through clinical disease history retrospection, doctors can gain experience and improve work quality.

5.2　Medical teaching　TCM inpatient record is very precious and vivid teaching materials. Through writing and reading TCM inpatient record, doctors and medical students can combine medical theory and clinical practice closely, thus consolidating what have learned and expanding their horizon. Ultimately, doctors' and medical students' thinking ability can be extraordinarily enhanced and the style of health care can be greatly improved.

5. 3 **Scientific research**　TCM inpatient record is the main material in clinical research. Through summarizing clinical records, doctors constantly seek objective principles in disease onset, development and therapeutic prognosis. Aiming at studying the relationship between clinical treatment, preventive measures, and disease, rehabilitation, advanced medical technologies and drugs have been discovered and filtrated, thereby promoting medical career to continuously develop.

5. 4　**Hospital management**　Vast data from TCM inpatient record could objectively reflect hospital management level such as hospital condition, technique quality, medical service quality, management measures and medical ethics. Therefore, through checking and analyzing record, it is a good way to realize hospital condition, improve medical service quality, enhance hospital management and increase hospital management level.

5. 5　**Disease prevention**　Through classified statistic and analysis, doctors and hospital can know development situations of common diseases and frequently-occurring diseases, providing evidence to disease prevention.

5. 6　**Legislation**　TCM inpatient record is legal basis in dealing with medical negligence and medical disputes. Therefore, TCM inpatient record can protect patients' and doctors' legitimate rights and interests.

6. Suggesting Reading After Class

6. 1　Zhu W, Zhu J. Chinese and western medica uniform format-management problems and counter measures [J]. Modern Hospital, 2014, 14(10): 96.

6. 2　Record writing editorial committee. Fundamental Norms of Record Writing (2010 version) [S]. Beijing: People's Medical Publishing House, 2010.

7. Homework

22 years old Female

Chief complaint: recurrent palpitation for 1 month.

History: 1 month ago, without any reason, had palpitation, mild, without chest pain. No syncope, no dyspnea, no lower limb swelling, no trembling arms, no fever, normal appetite. With night sweating, flushed cheeks, thirst with desire to drink, scanty yellow urine, dry stool, reddish tongue with scanty fluid, thin and rapid pulse.

No communicable disease history, allergic to seafood.

Unmarried, normal menstruation.

After taking history from SP patient, please write a inpatient record.

References

[1] Centers for Medicare & Medicaid Services. Personal Health Records [EB/OL]. [2012 − 04 − 14]. https://www.cms.gov/Medicare/E-Health/PerHealthRecords.

第七章

中医临床案例报告书写

　　中医学理论的建立和完成来源于长期临床实践。病例报告是一个不可替代的形式,它记录了生动实用的病例的诊断、治疗原则、治疗方法、治疗效果和预后。它充分体现了中医理论与临床实际的结合。

　　因此,病例报告具有继承和交流临床经验的作用,是中医理论发展的重要组成部分。

　　针对一个或一组患者的病例报告和病例系列研究非常适用于中医,因为中医强调个体化治疗。即使诊断为同一种疾病的患者很可能会接受不同的治疗,这是个体化的体现。不同的中医师有可能为同一患者开出不同的方剂成分和剂量。而读者能从中医药病例报告中参考治疗措施,应用于临床实践。病例报告是关于患者如何被诊断,以及为什么要进行特定的干预的记录。

　　许多中医著作记载的病例,长期以来在中医理论的发展中承担了一个重要的角色,如《伤寒杂病论》《临证指南医案》《名医类案》等。书写病例报告是中医临床实践记录的关键。

一、定义

　　1. 病例报告　指单个病例报告,也称个案报道,就是对单个患者接受治疗措施后产生的结果进行描述和评价。

　　2. 病例系列　是对一批患者接受治疗措施后的临床结果进行描述和评价。病例系列报告按时间不同分为回顾性病例报告和前瞻性病例报告。

二、如何写案例报告

(一)中医临床医师为什么要写病例报告

1. 对于过去　一个病例报告可能是唯一公布的记录,在一个给定的临床情况下,治疗和干预措施的记录。

2. 对于现在 能告诉其他中医师相关的治疗方法。作为一种可能的干预措施治疗疾病。

3. 对于未来 案例系列报告,有助于进一步指出中医临床研究的方向,提供更可靠的临床证据。

（二）病例从哪里来

（1）从您接诊的患者：新的疾病或条件/罕见疾病报告/常见病的特殊表现。

（2）从医师自己：新的或独特的治疗方法。

（3）后续结果：意想不到的疗效/意想不到的并发症的发生或处理。

（三）如何选择案例报告

（1）您选择的情况应该是有趣的案例,并对其他中医医师有借鉴意义。

（2）你选择的案例不应该在文献中以前有过报道(这意味着你需要做一个文献检索)。

（3）您选择的情况应该是完整的;你应该在文件记录中有足够的信息。

（四）接下来您该做什么

（1）找到您可能想要写的案例,以及预期的读者。

（2）检索杂志社是否允许病例报告,并彻底阅读作者指导。

（3）阅读其中的几本杂志,学习已发表的文章写法。

三、病例报告结构

（1）标题。

（2）摘要：介绍或文献综述目前研究的治疗。

（3）病例报告：患者信息及描述、治疗计划和治疗结果。

（4）讨论：讨论结果的影响、案件的不足、对未来研究的建议。

（5）结论。

（6）致谢(如需要)。

（7）参考文献(书籍,文学)。

（8）参考数据(CT、X 射线、胸腔镜检查、组织学)。

（9）详细内容见图 7 - 1、图 7 - 2 和表 7 - 1。

结节病唾液腺受累为罕见的表现形式
病例报告

前言 结节病是一种不明原因的多系统疾病，其特征在于受累器官中存在非干酪性肉芽肿。在90%的病例中，肺部受到影响。诊断后，有30%的患者无症状，胸部放射线检查发现偶然异常，常见的肺外表现可见于皮肤、眼睛、血管内皮、肌肉组织。肾脏、心脏、腺体、中枢神经系统也可能受累。

目标 基于病例报道描述结节病的少见表现。

方法 临床资料及文献回顾。

结果 作者报告了26岁女性，既往高血压、鼻窦炎、肥胖，表现出双侧唾液腺无痛性肿大。

症状：口干、乏力、无明显呼吸困难或咳嗽。

查体

• 皮肤无异常。

• 肺部查体阴性。

实验室检查

• 红细胞沉降率增快，血管紧张素转换酶（ACE）升高。

• 红细胞、白细胞计数正常。

• 肾功能正常。

• 免疫相关检查无异常。

唾液腺活检：非干酪样肉芽肿。

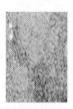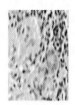

胸片及胸部CT：双侧肺门增大。

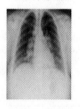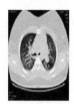

镓核素扫描未查。

结论 病例特点，ACE升高及唾液腺活检非干酪样肉芽肿，符合结节病唾液腺受累表现。患者活动耐受力降低及乏力，并表现为会自发缓解唾液腺增大。因此，皮质类固醇疗法的应用仍然暂时为使用。

参考文献 略。

图7-1 结节病唾液腺受累为罕见的表现形式病例报告

标题： 1例充血性心力衰竭继发单纯性胸腔积液的中药方治疗成功案例

摘要

目的 病例阐述了中药复方治疗充血性心力衰竭（CHF）后单侧胸腔积液的潜在疗效。

主题 一位79岁女性单侧胸膜腔积液2年。胸腔积液分析未发现感染、肺结核或恶性肿瘤。她接受了慢性心力衰竭的常规治疗，但症状仍然存在。因此，她寻求作者的中医诊所帮助。

干预以及结果 这个患者采用生脉散、泻白散、葶苈子等中药颗粒剂，每日3次，共4周。每日剂量根据患者的临床反应和随访的胸部X线检查进行调整。治疗8个月后，症状改善，胸腔积液明显改善。

结论 在常规治疗反应不佳时，提示中药复方对预防CHF继发单侧胸腔积液的发生有重要作用，并且对中医药物作用机制的研究是有必要的。

前言　胸膜腔积液是胸腔内液体积留的结果，表明存在肺、胸膜或肺外疾病。尽管许多不同的疾病可能导致胸腔积液，但在美国，最常见的病因是 CHF、肺炎和癌症。心脏病的总体发病率参考鹿特丹—项以人群为基础的研究中，心力衰竭的发生率估计为 3.9％，随着年龄的增长而迅速增加。欧洲学会指南认为，心力衰竭是一种病理生理状态，具有以下特征：症状（呼吸急促或疲劳，休息或运动时踝关节肿胀）以及心脏功能不全。由于肺毛细血管压力升高，肺间质液体增加，导致胸腔积液和肺水肿，导致劳累性呼吸困难。心力衰竭相关的积液通常是双侧的，如果是单侧积液，则应进行胸腔穿刺（可能对利尿剂治疗无效）。大约 75％ 的充血性心力衰竭在开始利尿后 48 小时内消退。然而，仍有一些病例对常规治疗或胸腔穿刺无效。在中医观念中，治疗难治性胸腔积液有多种策略，包括中药方剂、针灸和食疗。本病例报告一位因充血性心力衰竭而出现单侧胸腔积液的患者，在 8 个月的随访期内，成功地用中药治疗……

　　病例报告　一位 79 岁的妇女，她年轻时健康状况一直很好，直到 20 年前，她开始咳嗽，并严重呼吸困难。她最初的胸部平片显示右侧有单侧胸腔积液。胸腔穿刺术后的胸腔积液分析未发现其他细菌感染或恶性肿瘤，怀疑其继发于 CHF 的单侧胸腔积液。她接受了常规的利尿剂治疗，症状改善。然而，同样的情况在 2010 年 3 月再次出现，这次她的胸部平片显示左侧胸膜腔积液……

中药配方的作用及适应证

中文名	功　　效	适　应　证
生脉散	补气，养阴，复脉，止汗	心力衰竭、冠心病、慢性肺源性心脏病的气阴两虚，表现为大量出汗、口渴、气短、干咳、乏力、心悸、心律不齐、口干、舌red不多、脉细弱
泻白散	清肺，止咳平喘，养胃	肺热，引起咳嗽、哮喘、午后发热、口渴、自汗、唇颊红肿、面颊红肿、舌红、脉搏加快
葶苈子	宣肺，平喘，化饮，消肿	肺积水，哮喘，胸胁饮停，痰浊咳嗽，肺脓肿

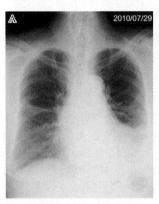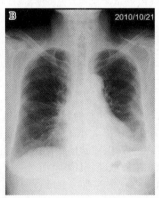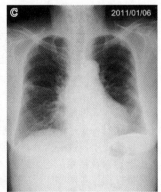

胸部平片系列。A. 首次就诊。B. 3 个月后。C. 6 个月后。左侧单侧胸膜积液经中药治疗后逐渐消退

讨论 本报告中的患者被诊断为 CHF 继发的复发性单侧胸腔积液。2010 年 3 月至 6 月,她接受了利尿剂常规治疗,并接受了 3 次胸腔穿刺。因为胸腔积液没有自然消退,她选择了中医药治疗。在台湾,中医医生通常会根据患者的症状,开浓缩草药颗粒。草药颗粒是按照 GMP 标准加工和浓缩的纯生草药混合物制备的过程。不像研磨而成的中药粉,其提取物颗粒不仅含有相同的成分,而且还保留了传统……

图 7-2 1 例充血性心力衰竭继发单纯性胸腔积液的中药方治疗成功案例

表 7-1 病例报告结构

条 目	编号	描 述
标题	1	1)标题中需要提及"病例报道"或者类似术语(如:病例记录,或病例研究) 2)如果时候病例系列,需要包含病例/患者数量
摘要	2	1)简述本病例的独特之处,及其讨论要点和评价 2)包括:主要症状、类证鉴别、治疗措施、结果评估、病例亮点
关键词	3	病例相关的主要要点,3~5 个关键词,如:病例报道,病名,证型,治疗
引言	4	1)为什么选择这例病例做报道 2)来自患者或监护人的知情同意书 3)关于目前诊疗及既往研究的文献综述 4)用陈述的方式撰写病例
患者信息	5	1)列出患者信息(性别,年龄,就诊日期,节气) 2)建议包括患者的体重、身高、婚姻情况、职业、病例来源(就诊医院、住院或门诊病例),治疗和报道病例的医生职称
临床发现	6	1)描述主诉 2)现病史 3)中医证候 4)舌脉特点 5)选择性内容:过敏史,社会生活史,家族史,遗传史
诊断	7	1)中医诊断:必须包括辨证,诊断标准需要引用参考文献 2)现代医学诊断:包括检查结果,诊断标准需要引用参考文献,以及鉴别诊段
治疗	8	1)中医治则 2)中药处方 a.药物名称,剂量,使用方式,治程,药物产地 b.建议报告药物质控情况 3)针灸治疗 a.穴位名、取穴位置、单侧/双侧、操作(进针角度、深度、手法、针具类型、留针时间、治疗频次) b.电针参数 c.艾灸数量
结果评估	9	1)使用广泛认可的金标准评估 2)如果使用自拟标准需要有详尽的备注说明
随访	10	1)在治疗期间,药物变换的依据 2)随访时间及结果 3)患者的起居、饮食、情绪及环境

（续表）

条　目	编号	描　　述
讨论	11	1）说明本病例诊断或治疗的意义和困难 2）鉴别诊断 3）阐述处方的基本治则以及本案例中的"重点"信息 4）讨论对结果的影响因素 5）讨论病例在现有文献中的含义和相关性 6）病例报告中的局限性 7）对未来研究的建议
致谢	12	1）对本案有贡献的人致谢
参考文献	13	1）本案例相关的引用文献（如果期刊对参考文献数量要求）
图表	14	1）本案例相关的图表

四、写作建议

（1）准确，简介，凝练。

（2）了解你的读者或杂志。你需要通过回顾过去在杂志上发表的案例报告类型及其"作者须知"页面，以读者和杂志为目标。如果有疑问，您可以联系您正在考虑的杂志的编辑人员，在写作开始之前讨论。

（3）使用主要参考资料。主要来源是原始材料，提供直接证据或由实际参与活动的人创建的第一手记录。这些资料是你解释分析病例以及得出你的结论的宝贵依据。

（4）在罕见病中选择评述类文章。文献回顾是病例报告最重要的基石。特别是因为早期只有罕见病例被视为病例报告发表。因此，要确定该病例的罕见性，必须彻底做到回顾文献。

（5）避免指责或点评其他作者观点。

（6）确保患者的隐私。

（7）牢记"准确""简介""凝练"的原则。

五、如何将文献发表

提高杂志接受论文的因素。

（1）获得书面知情同意和保密同意。

（2）根据你文章要表达的信息，选择你的目标读者和杂志。

（3）在写作前和编者讨论你想法。

（4）有条件的话，与相关专家协作讨论内容。

（5）避免过于详尽的文献回顾。

（6）尽可能简洁明了。

六、阅读材料

1. Cohen H. How to write a patient case report［J］. American Journal of Health-System Pharmacy，2006，63（19）：1888－92.

2. Chelvarajah R，Bycroft J. Writing and publishing case reports：the road to success ［J］. Acta Neurochirurgica，2004，146（3）：313.

3. White A. Writing case reports — author guidelines for acupuncture in medicine［J］. Acupuncture in Medicine Journal of the British Medical Acupuncture Society，2004，22（2）：83.

4. Martyn C. Case reports，case series and systematic reviews.［J］. Qjm Monthly Journal of the Association of Physicians，2002，95（4）：197－198.

5. Brodell R T. Do more than discuss that unusual case. Write it up！［J］. Postgraduate Medicine，2000，108（2）：19－20，23.

6. Yang H，Fei YT，Liu JP. Reporting methods for clinical cases on Chinese medicine and experts' experiences-design of case report.［J］Tradition Chin Med（Chin），2008（49）：215－217.

七、课后习题

选择一个病例书写病例报道。

参考文献

［1］The Lancet Haematology. About the lancet haematology［EB/OL］.［2021－01－05］. https://www.thelancet.com/lanhae/about.

［2］李汉道,许秀莲.中草药治疗充血性心力衰竭继发单侧胸腔积液 1 例[J].替代医学杂志,2012,18(5)：509－512.

［3］秋和久永,斋藤,福田英彦,等.康宝方治疗阻塞性睡眠呼吸暂停综合征 1 例[J].精神病学与临床神经科学,1999,53(2)：303－305.

Chapter Seven

TCM Case Report Writing

TCM theory is to establish and complete long-term from clinical practice. Case report is an irreplaceable form of report that records the diagnosis, treatment principles, treatment methods, treatment effects and prognosis of vivid and practical cases. It fully embodies the combination of TCM theory and clinical practice.

Therefore, case report has the function of inheriting and exchanging clinical experience and is an important part of the development of TCM theory.

Case reports and case series studies for one or a group of patients are well suited for TCM because TCM emphasizes individualized treatment. Even patients diagnosed with the same disease are likely to receive different treatments, which is an embodiment of individualization. Different TCM doctors may prescribe different prescription ingredients and doses for the same patient. Readers can refer to treatments from TCM case reports for clinical practice. The case report is a record of how the patient was diagnosed and why a specific intervention was to be performed.

The cases recorded in many TCM works have played an important role in the development of TCM theory for a long time, such as the theory of typhoid fever, the clinical case of clinical trials, and the case of famous doctors. Writing a case report is the key to the clinical practice record of TCM.

1. Definition

Case report is a detailed report of the symptoms, signs, diagnosis, treatments, and follow-ups of an individual patient. Case reports may contain a demographic profile of the patient, but usually describe an unusual or novel occurrence. Some case reports also contain a literature review of other reported cases.

Case series is a type of medical research study that tracks subjects with a known exposure, such as patients who have received a similar treatment, or examines their medical records for exposure and outcome. Case series may be consecutive or non-consecutive, depending on whether all cases presenting to the reporting authors over a period were included, or only a selection. The case series is divided into retrospective, prospective, and time series case reports based on time order. The concept of exposure and outcomes come from epidemiology. Epidemiological studies are aimed, where possible, at revealing unbiased relationships between exposures such as alcohol or smoking, biological agents, stress, or chemicals to mortality or morbidity. The identification of causal relationships between these exposures and outcomes is an important aspect of epidemiology.

2. How to begin

2.1 Why should you do this

2.1.1 For past: A case report may be the published evidence on an intervention in a given clinical situation.

2.1.2 For present: You might tell other doctors regarding the therapy as a possible intervention.

2.1.3 For future: Research, even case reports, helps to point the way to further research on the topic leading to more reliable evidence.

2.2 Where to start

2.2.1 From your patient: New disease or condition/rare or sparsely reported/unusual presentation of a common condition

2.2.2 From doctor yourself : New or unique treatment.

Eg: Shen SY, Yao CH, Fu YT, et al. Acupuncture as complementary therapy for hypoxic encephalopathy: a case study [J]. Complementary Therapies in Medicine, 2010, 18(6): 265 - 268.

2.2.3 From follow-up: Unexpected outcome for one condition when treating for another condition/Unexpected complication during treatment

Eg: Lord GM, Tagore R, Cook T, et al. Nephropathy caused by Chinese herbs in the UK [J]. Lancet, 1999, 354(9177): 481.

PS: The case report is based on the clinical practice record (Outpatient record, Inpatient record, etc). It is the "start" of a good case report that collecting, reviewing, and analyzing your clinical cases.

2.3 How to choose a case to report

2.3.1 The case you choose should be interesting to other doctors.

2.3.2 The case you choose should not be previously numerous represented in the literature (that means you need to do a literature search).

2.3.3 The case you choose should be complete. You should have enough information in the file to present the case (including patient consent form, audio/video material, photo, etc).

2.4 What should you do next

Deciding which case to report should not be an insurmountable barrier. Different journals publish different kinds of cases. Some may be looking for originality; others consider the educational value and usefulness for the reader to be more important than uniqueness. You need to target your audience and journal by reviewing what types of case reports have been published in the journal in the past and their "instructions to authors" pages. If in doubt, you may want to contact the editorial staff of the journal you are considering to discuss your intentions before starting.

It is essential that you obtain written consent from the patient's family and the patient. Some journals now have their own consent forms, which have to be completed by the patient or parent. Some cases benefit from a photograph.

2.4.1 Find a case that you might want to write up.

2.4.2 Determine your audience.

2.4.3 Check to see if journals allow case report and read the instruction for Authors thoroughly.

2.4.4 Look at a few journals that focus on this audience and read their instructions to authors.

2.4.5 Read several case reports from that journal.

Eg: http://www.thelancet.com/lanres/about.

http://www.thelancet.com/pb/assets/raw/Lancet/authors/tlrm-info-for-authors-may-2017.pdf.

3. How to structure the report

Start with a brief abstract and a list of key words. The case description follows, and should contain the essential details and relevant test results, with normal values in parentheses. The discussion section comes next. The theme should be your educational message. Cite the literature only as needed to make your point; do not present your entire literature review. A review article is very different from a case report. Highlight the significance of what you are presenting and what you learn clearly and briefly! End with a summary or conclusions paragraph, which is generally your "take-home message".

3.1 Introduction

3.1.1 An introduction or literature review on the presenting condition and previously studied treatments.

3.1.2 Describe case in narrative form.

3.2 Case report/summary

3.2.1 A description of the patient.

3.2.2 The treatment plan and results of treatment.

3.3 Discussion

3.3.1 Discussion of the implications of the outcomes.

3.3.2 Describe implications and relevance of case in the context of current literature.

3.3.3 Limitation of the case report.

3.3.4 Suggestions for future studies.

3.4 Conclusion

3.5 Acknowledgements (if applicable).

3.6 References(book, literature).

3.7 Tables, figures(CT, X-ray, thoracoscopy, histology).

SARCOIDOSIS – SALIVARY GLAND INVOLVEMENT AS AN UNCOMMON PRESENTATION FORM
CASE REPORT

Diana Fernandes, Clara Brito, Pedro Soares, Luisa Teixeira, Sheila Arroja, Renato Saraiva

Hospital Santo André, E.P.E. – Leira, Portugal

Introduction:

Sarcoidosis is a multisystem disease of unknown cause, which is characterized by noncaseous granuloma in the affected organs. In 90% of cases, the lungs are affected. After diagnosis, 30% of patients were asymptomatic. Rare abnormalities were found in chest radiography. Common extrapulmonary manifestations were found in skin, eyes, vascular endothelium and muscle tissue. The kidneys, heart, glands and central nervous system may also be involved.

Objectives:

Description of rare manifestations of sarcoidosis based on case reports

Material and Methods:

Clinical data and literature review

Results:

A 26 year old female with previous hypertension, sinusitis and obesity showed painless swelling of bilateral salivary glands.

Symptom:
• Dry mouth
• Weakness
• No obvious dyspnea or cough

Physical examination:
• No skin abnormality
• Lung examination was negative

Laboratory inspection:
• Erythrocyte sedimentation rate increased rapidly and angiotensin converting enzyme level increased
• Red blood cell and white blood cell counts were normal
• Normal renal function
• There was no abnormality in immune related examination.

Salivary gland biopsy: non caseous granuloma

Chest X-ray and CT: bilateral hilar enlargement.

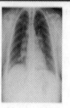 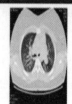

Gallium isotope scan failed

Conclusions:

Case characteristics: elevated Angiotensin converting enzyme level and noncaseous granuloma in salivary gland biopsy were consistent with the manifestations of salivary gland involvement in sarcoidosis. The patient's activity tolerance decreased and fatigue, and showed spontaneous remission and enlargement of salivary gland. Therefore, the application of corticosteroid therapy is still temporary.

Reference:

• Lynch JP 3rd, Ma YL, Koss MN,White ES.Pulmonary sarcoidosis.Semin Respir Crit Care Med.2007;28:53-74.
•Baughman RP, Lower EE, du Bois RM.Sarcoidosis.Lancet2003; 361:1 111
•Thomas KW, Hunninghake GW, Sarcoidosis. JAMA 2003; 289:3300

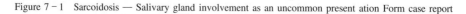

Figure 7 – 1　Sarcoidosis — Salivary gland involvement as an uncommon present ation Form case report

THE JOURNAL OF ALTERNATIVE AND COMPLEMENTARY MEDICINE
Volume 18, Number 5, 2012, pp. 509–512
⊕ Mary Ann Liebert, Inc.
DOI: 10.1089/acm.2011.0292

Case Report

A Case of Unilateral Pleural Effusion Secondary to Congestive Heart Failure Successfully Treated with Traditional Chinese Herbal Formulas

Han-Dao Lee, MD,[1] and Hsien-Hsueh Elley Chiu, MD[1,2]

Abstract

Objectives: A case is presented that illustrates the potential effect of traditional Chinese medicine (TCM) herbal formulas on treatment for unilateral pleural effusion secondary to congestive heart failure (CHF).
Subject: A 79-year-old woman experienced episodic dyspnea with unilateral pleural effusion for 2 years. Thoracocentesis with pleural fluid analysis revealed no infection, tuberculosis, or malignancy. She had received conventional treatment for CHF but the symptoms persisted. Therefore, she visited the authors' TCM clinic for help.
Interventions and outcome: This patient was treated with TCM herbal granules including Shengmaisan, Xiebaisan, and Tinglizi, 3 times a day for 4 weeks. The daily dosage was adjusted on the basis of the patient's clinical response and her follow-up chest X-ray studies. After 8 months of treatment, her symptoms improved and the pleural effusion showed significant regression.
Conclusions: It is suggested that TCM herbal formulas could play an important role in preventing the progression of unilateral pleural effusion secondary to CHF, in case of poor response to conservative treatment. Additional studies about the mechanism of action of the medication involved are warranted.

Introduction

A pleural effusion is the result of fluid accumulation in the pleural space, which indicates the presence of pulmonary, pleural, or extrapulmonary disease. Although many different diseases may cause a pleural effusion, the most common causes in the United States are congestive heart failure (CHF), pneumonia, and cancer. The overall prevalence of heart failure in a population-based Rotterdam study was estimated at 3.9%, which increases rapidly with age. According to the guidelines of the European Society of Cardiology, heart failure is a pathophysiologic state with the following features: symptoms (e.g shortness of breath or fatigue, at rest or during exercise, ankle swelling) and objective evidence of cardiac dysfunction. Increased interstitial fluid in the lung due to elevated pulmonary capillary pressure leads to both pleural effusion and pulmonary edema, causing exertional breathlessness. Since CHF-related effusions are typically bilateral, thoracocentesis is indicated if effusion is seen unilaterally or has not responded to diuretic therapy. Approximately 75% of effusions due to CHF resolve within 48 hours after diuresis is begun. However, there are still some cases that do not respond to conventional therapy or thoracocentesis. In the Chinese medicine concept, there are several strategies of treating refractory pleural effusion, including herbal formula, acupuncture, and food therapy. This case report deals with a patient who had unilateral pleural effusion secondary to CHF and who was successfully treated with traditional Chinese medicine (TCM) herbal formulas over an 8-month follow-up period.

Case Report

A 79-year-old woman had been in good health until 2 years ago, when she started to have coughs and severe dyspnea on exertion. Her initial chest plain film study showed unilateral pleural effusion on the right side. The pleural fluid analysis after thoracocentesis revealed neither bacterial infection nor malignancy. Unilateral pleural effusion secondary to CHF was suspected. She was treated conservatively with diuretic pills and the symptoms subsided. However, the same situation recurred in March 2010. This time her chest plain film study showed left-side pleural effusion.

Table 2 Function and Indication of Traditional Chinese Medicine Herbal Formula

Chinese names	Function	Indication
Shengmaisan	• Tonify Qi • Nourish Yin • Stimulate pulse • Prevent excessive sweating	Qi-Yin deficiency in heart failure, coronary artery disease, and chronic pulmonary-heart disease, with symptoms of profuse sweating, thirst, shortness of breath, dry cough, fatigue, palpitations, irregular heartbeats, dry mouth, red Tongue without much saliva, and a weak and thready pulse
Xiebaisan	• Clear lung heat • Relieve asthma and cough • Nourish the stomach	Lung heat has damaged Yin, causing cough, asthma, fever rising in the afternoon, thirst, spontaneous sweating, red lips and cheeks, facial edema, red Tongue, and rapid pulse.
Tinglizi	• Purge the lung • Relieve asthma • Promote water metabolism • Disperse swelling	Asthma due to water retention in the lungs, water distention in the chest and ribs, cough due to the retention of phlegm and fluid, pulmonary abscess

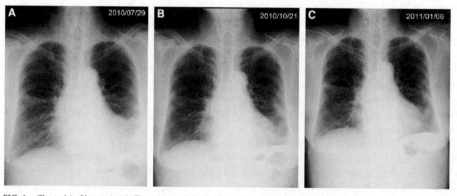

FIG. 1. Chest plain films series. **A.** First visit to clinic. **B.** Three (3) months later. **C.** Six (6) months later. Unilateral pleural effusion on the left side gradually subsided after treatment with Traditional Chinese Medicine herbal formulas.

Discussion

The patient in this report was diagnosed with recurrent unilateral pleural effusion secondary to CHF. During March to June in 2010, she had been treated conservatively with diuretics and received thoracocentesis 3 times. Because there was no spontaneous regression of pleural fluids, she chose alternative TCM treatment.

In Taiwan, TCM doctors usually preferred to prescribe concentrated herbal granules with formulas plus a specific single herb according to the patient's symptoms. The herbal granules were prepared with an all-raw herbal mixture cooked and concentrated following GMP standard process. Unlike ground herbal powders, the extract granules not only retain the same ingredients and the spirit of traditional herbal decoction, but also have been screened from pesticides.

References

1. McGrath EE, Blades Z, Needham J, Anderson PB. A systematic approach to the investigation and diagnosis of a unilateral pleural effusion. Intern J Clin Pract 2009; 63: 1653 – 1659.
2. Light RW. Clinical practice. Pleural effusion. NEJM 2002; 346: 1971 – 1977.
3. Mosterd A, Hoes AW, de Bruyne MC, et al. Prevalence of heart failure and left ventricular dysfunction in the general population: The Rotterdam study. Eur Heart J 1999; 20: 447 – 455.
4. Task Force for the Diagnosis and Treatment of Chronic Heart Failure, European Society of Cardiology: Remme WJ, Swedberg K. Guidelines for the diagnosis and treatment of chronic heart failure. Eur Heart J 2001; 22: 1527 – 1560.
5. Puri S, Baker BL, Oakley CM, et al. Increased alveolar/capillary membrane resistance to gas transfer in patients with chronic heart failure. Br Heart J 1994; 72: 140 – 144.
6. Porcel JM. Pleural effusions from congestive heart failure. Semin Respir Crit Care Med 2010; 31: 689 – 697.
7. Porcel JM, Light RW. Diagnostic approach to pleural effusion in adults. Am Fam Physician 2006; 73: 1211 – 1220.

Figure 7 – 2   A case of unilateral pleural effusion secondary to congestive heart failure successfully treated with Traditional Chinese herbal formillas

Table 7 – 1   TCM case report recommendations for details

Item name	No	Brief description
Title	1	A. The word "case report" or similar terms (eg: medical record or case study) should appear in the title B. The number of cases/patients included if for case series
Abstract	2	A. Briefly describe the characteristics of the reporting cases, and state the discussion and comment B. a. main symptoms b. differentiation of disease and pattern c. treatment d. outcome assessment e. highlights of this case

(**continued**)

Item name	No	Brief description
Keywords	3	A. Key elements of this case in 3 – 5 words. Eg: case report, name of disease, name of pattern, treatment remedy
Introduction	4	A. Why choose this case to report B. The informed consent obtained from patients or their guardians C. Literature review on the presenting condition and previously studied treatments D. Describe case in narrative form
Patient information	5	A. List out patient's information (gender, age, date of consultation, the 24 solar terms) B. Recommend to report the patient's weight/height/marital status/occupation/source (name of hospital, inpatient, outpatient case), and the qualification of doctor who treat and report the case
Clinical Finding	6	A. Describe the main complaint B. Present medical history C. TCM symptoms and signs D. Characteristics on tongue and pulse E. Optional items include allergies, social life history, family/inheritance history

Diagnosis	7	A. For case diagnosed by TCM
		  a. Must report the differentiation of TCM patterns
		  b. Diagnostic criteria can be presented by citing related literatures
		B. For case diagnosed by modern medicine
		  a. Report examination findings
		  b. Diagnostic criteria can be presented by citing related literatures
		  c. Report the differential diagnosis

Treatment	8	A. The therapeutic principle of TCM
		B. Chinese herbal intervention
		  a. The product name, dosing, administration and treatment course, the place of cultivation
		  b. Recommend: report the quality control standard
		C. Acupuncture and moxibustion intervention
		  a. Acupoint name, location, uni/bilateral, operating procedure (insertion angle, depth, manipulation, needle type and retention time, and treatment frequencies).
		  b. Electroacupuncture parameter
		  c. Moxibustion units

Outcome assessment	9	A. Using widely recognized gold standard assessment criteria B. If applicable or self-designated criteria with explanation in detail
Follow-up	10	A. During the treatment period, the changes of treatment remedies with underlying rationale B. Follow-up visit with date and consequent, if applicable C. What patient had done: About diet, emotions and living, environment
Comments or Discussion	12	A. Specify the significances and difficulties for the diagnosis or treatment of this case B. Differential diagnosis C. Elaborate the rationale of prescription and the "take away" message from this case D. Discussion of the implications of the outcomes E. Describe implications and relevance of case in the context of current literature F. Limitation of the case report G. Suggestions for future studies

(continued)

Item name	No	Brief description
Acknowledgement	13	Acknowledge anyone who contributed towards this case
References	14	The literatures are relevant to this case (if it is limited with exact number of references)
Figure/Tables	15	The figures and tables are relevant to this case

4. General Tips

4.1 A = accuracy、B = brevity、C = clarity.

4.2 Know your audience/journal. You need to target your audience and journal by reviewing what types of case reports have been published in the journal in the past and their 'instructions to authors' pages. If in doubt, you may want to contact the editorial staff of the journal you are considering to discuss your intentions before starting.

4.3 Use primary references. Primary sources are original materials that provide direct evidence or firsthand records created by people who actually participated in an event. Such sources are invaluable tools for developing your own interpretations and reaching your own conclusions.

4.4 Select review articles in rare cases. Literature review has been the most important cornerstone of a case report. Especially since earlier only rare cases were considered as case reports. So to establish the rarity of the case it was important to thoroughly review the literature.

4.5 Avoid finger-pointing.

4.6 Ensure patient privacy.

4.7 Remember the ABCs of writing.

5. How to Maximize the Chance of Publication

Factors that enhance the chance of manuscript acceptance:

5.1 Obtain written, informed consent and maintain confidentiality.

5.2 Target audience or journal according to your message.

5.3 Consider discussing ideas with the editorial staff before starting.

5.4 Collaborate with a content expert, if appropriate.

5.5   Avoid an exhaustive literature review.

5.6   Aim for brevity and clarity.

These factors are particularly important in producing a manuscript which will be accepted for publication and summarized. They have been dealt with in the preceding sections of the present paper. An additional key issue arises when criticisms or a rejection is received from a journal after the paper has been submitted. Almost all case reports will require revisions as suggested by the peer reviewers. Address each point carefully and clearly with an accompanying letter explaining the changes. Do not take rejection personally because it does not necessarily reflect the quality of your report. You may need to target your audience a bit more carefully with your resubmission. If your case report is very brief or is rejected in its current format, you may consider resubmitting it as a letter to the editor.

6. Suggesting Reading

6.1   Cohen H. How to write a patient case report[J]. American journal of health-system pharmacy, 2006, 63(19): 1888 – 92.

6.2   Chelvarajah R, Bycroft J. Writing and publishing case reports: the road to success [J]. Acta Neurochirurgica, 2004, 146(3): 313.

6.3   White A. Writing case reports — author guidelines for acupuncture in medicine [J]. Acupuncture in Medicine Journal of the British Medical Acupuncture Society, 2004, 22 (2): 83.

6.4   Martyn C. Case reports, case series and systematic reviews.[J]. Qjm Monthly Journal of the Association of Physicians, 2002, 95(4): 197 – 8.

6.5   Brodell RT. Do more than discuss that unusual case. Write it up! [J]. Postgraduate Medicine, 2000, 108(2): 19 – 20, 23.

6.6   Yang H, Fei YT, Liu JP. Reporting methods for clinical cases on Chinese medicine and experts' experiences-d esign of case report.[J]. Tradition Chin Med (Chin), 2008(49): 215 – 217.

7. Assignment

You can choose a clinical case which is significant for clinical physicians to write a case report by yourself.

References

[1] The Lancet Haematology. About the lancet haematology [EB/OL]. [2021 - 01 - 05]. https://www.thelancet.com/lanhae/about.

[2] Lee HD, Chiu HH. A case of unilateral pleural effusion secondary to congestive heart failure successfully treated with traditional Chinese herbal formulas [J]. Altern Complement Med, 2012, 18(5). 509 - 512.

[3] Hisanaga A, Saitoh O, Fukuda H, et al. Treatment of obstructive sleep apnea syndrome with a Kampo-formula, San'o-shashin-to: a case report [J]. Psychiatry & Clinical Neurosciences, 1999, 53(2). 303 - 305.

第八章　中医平行病历的书写

　　病历，是医师对每位患者从疾病的发生、发展、转归，辅助检查、诊断、治疗方案等一系列医疗活动过程的记录。疾病和疼痛是两个不同的世界。前者是医护人员的世界，后者是患者的世界。诊疗过程中医护人员着眼于治疗、观察及记录疾病，而患者是体验和叙述病痛；医护人员身处寻找病因与病理指标的客观世界，患者却身处诉说身体和心灵痛苦所经历的主观世界。

　　现代医学并不能解决所有问题，有时是治愈，常常是安慰。为了与患者拉近信任的距离，建立医患之间的大爱，培养医患情感的共同体，医务工作者可以掌握书写平行病历的方法来达到医师医疗判断和共情能力的双重提升。

一、定义

　　平行病历，又称"叙事医学病历"，是医护人员在书写临床标准病历之外，用非技术性语言书写患者的疾苦和体验。通过叙事医学病历的书写，可以有效整合、思考和升华平时的医务工作，有助于更好地实践如何共情患者的疾苦。前面第2~第4章节学习的标准的临床病历是一种格式化病历，与平行病历是一个故事的两种讲法。中医药是非常注重疾病治疗中的人文关怀的，中医诊病注重患者的身体疾苦与精神情志及人生境遇的关系。在《素问·疏五过论篇》中论述的"五过"，即指诊治疾病时易犯的五种过失，包括因忽视患者的社会地位变迁、思想情绪变化、精神内伤状况和患病的始末过程以及不明诊脉的原则，而发生误诊与误治的五种过失，明确了心理、社会的致病因素，强调"病从内生"、心身合一的病因病机。而这种情况以平行病历形式描述更易于理解。

　　平行病历是指在临床环节中要求医学生或年轻医师为同一位患者准备两份病历：一份是标准的临床病历，是记录客观的、被观察的生理、病理指征。医生处在寻找病因与病理指标的客观世界,这是被观察、记录的世界。另一份是平行病历,是由医师书写的患者叙述和体验的疾苦,是患者的故事以及自我的人文观察与反应,是主观的、被叙述的人格、人性故事,隐藏在患者的疾痛故事中,包括疾病所赋予的社会、心理角色,所象征的意义、所带来的情感变化与所隐含的观念、信仰。

二、平行病历与格式化病历的区别

传统的格式化病历有一定的规则,顺序不能颠倒,以客观描述为基础,就事论事,不能随意引申,不可无根据猜测,病历书写中只要把病说清楚、讲明白,顺理成章地推出临床诊断,就算完成了病历记录的工作。写格式化病历时,医生是客观的,态度是冷静的,有确定的模板,不能随意突破。从主诉、现病史、既往史、个人史,无论在字数、顺序、用词,还是在症状的描述上都不能主观发挥,体现的是医生缜密的思维。而平行病历,侧重于医生对患者疾苦的关注,通过医生的共情将患者的经历与感受再现出来,进而把医生接纳到患者的共情圈里,医患双方携手共抗疾病。

平行病历中有感情的注入,再现了医患心灵的碰撞,体现了医学的人文价值。平行病历没有固定模式,书写时除了医学基本功,还需要有人文的包容度,更需要融入做人的情感。

平行病历的宗旨是与叙事医学一脉相承——通过对疾病的叙事化,将患者、疾病、病痛折磨联系起来,将疾病的生物学世界和人的生活世界联系起来,使疾病得到阐释并产生意义。

三、如何写平行病历

平行病历,简单理解就是"病"+"情":一边写病,一边写情。它是患者真实的疾病体验,患者既有疾病的表现,又有心理的压力,更有思想的困惑。它除了像传统的病历,给患者谈病痛的机会,还鼓励患者说出想说却不习惯、不敢说的"悄悄话"。医生要打开自己的"雷达",不光记录问出的东西,还要倾听患者的"言外之意",甚至主动去猜测患者的隐喻。平行病历是要求医者在格式化病历的严谨格式之外,也不能忽视感情,患者的七情六欲一定要了如指掌。

平行病历谈感情、聊心理,这需要文学的底蕴,需要哲学的思考,需要读经典,而且要读人文大家的书。写平行病历不需要故弄玄虚,不需要宣教、说大话,只要情真意切,即使没有什么轰轰烈烈的事件,仅凭真实生动的细节也能击中人心。

写平行病历能给予医师什么 平行病历的书写对于医师的职业生涯来说是很有意义

的。这使他们能在诊疗过程中切身关注患者的真实遭遇,提高从患者角度考虑问题的能力,这也是医疗训练中不可缺少的一部分。而中医学的医案医话恰恰是标准病历和平行病历结合的体现。建立在中医医案医话基础之上的中医平行病历,符合当前重视临床人文关怀的大背景、大环境,为当前医患双方提供了科学有效的沟通平台,医生通过沟通交流,并记录、共情、分享给更多的医者,甚至患者。平行病历的作用主要有以下几方面:书写平行病历,可以改善医师的职业倦怠感。因为它没有条框的约束,可以让你尽情地挥洒感情,借助形形色色的故事,让你排解出内心的压力与困惑。平行病历可以助医师发现患者对疾病的体验,这可能比化验数据、影像报告更有临床价值,对疾病救治和临床医学意义的理解更为有效。也给了医师对临床事物更多的反思机会。平行病历还让医师融入患者的境况,身临其境了解患者的感受。这使医师对今后患者的情况有预判并对自己未来将面临的疾病的苦痛、死亡的恐惧,有了充分的思考,也做了必要的心理准备。

训练有素的读者能与小说家心意相通,故事的叙述者与聆听者能够无间互动。借助文字,让医生与患者产生碰撞,进而达到心灵之间的交流,是重拾医学人文的一种方式。平行病历可使医师更谦逊、更尊重患者、更能够站在患者的立场思考问题,也能发现医师这份职业更深层的意义。

四、平行病历的书写要点

中医平行病历在古代医案和医话中已有相当多的体现。《丹溪翁传》:"一妇人产有物不上如衣裾,医不能喻。翁曰,此子宫也,气血虚,故随子而下。即与黄芪、当归之剂,而加升麻举之,仍用皮工之法,以五倍子作汤洗濯,皱其皮。少选,子宫上,翁慰之曰,三年后可再生儿,无忧也。如之。"这是名人传记节选,还并非标准的医案,但当时的记载除了写清何人何情用何药而愈,还记载了丹溪翁关注患者,心理安慰她"三年后还可以生育,不用担心"。一方面体现了医者仁心,另一方面也体现出当时的医案医话记载也非常重视人文关怀,体现医师和患者的互动。病例的书写并不是冷冰冰的对于疾病的描述和概括,还展露出医师对患者最真诚的关切以及由此给患者带来的喜悦和安慰。这样的描述方法就是中医叙事医学中的平行病历的书写方法,非常关注患者的感受。

在平行病历的文本当中,需关注一个细节即细读,实际上是在医师书写平行病历的时候通过文本的书写更加懂得患者的真实遭遇。也通过这个文本的细读,去审视自己在临床当中的心理变化和干预历程。

平行病历的三个重要的元素就是关注、再现和行动。关注就是关注那些情节,再现当时那个患病的情境,能够采取正确合理的行动使者得到更好的心境,帮助疾病的恢复。

五、平行病历的格式

（1）平行病历作为叙事医学书写格式，主要由五个部分组成：时间、情节、想象、共情（感觉/情感）、意义。

（2）中医平行病历的举例：以下是通过对中医古籍的研读和亲身参与的临床实践，写下的一份中医平行病历。

"2014年9月15日秋分，来门诊的一位中年女人，45岁，面色憔悴，胸中有异物感已经2个月，各种检查无果，在陈述自己病情的时候竟痛哭失声，越发觉得自己呼吸不畅。细细了解之后得知她的丈夫丢了工作，长期在家酗酒，对孩子也不关心。她一直是全职主妇，没有经济来源，也没有谋生能力，家中争吵是常有的事情。后来，她每次来看病都要倾诉很久，包括孩子最近是不是听话、成绩如何，说起孩子，她眼中闪出不一样的光亮，好似那就是她生命中的救命稻草。该患者舌质暗淡、苔薄白腻脉弦，中医诊断是'梅核气'，这个疾病除了中药疗法以外，心理疗法也尤为重要。用药这小半年患者自觉症状缓解，胸中舒畅很多，但并未痊愈，时有反复加重，每每与争吵和生闷气有关。后来经我再三研究她的病历和情况，除了药物、导引等治疗外，还给了她走出家门、走向社会、参与社会活动的建议，她采纳了。患者去了当地一个私人幼儿园帮厨，一方面缓解心中郁闷，一方面可以缓解家中的经济负担，约3个月后患者特地前来诊室，面带喜色向我致谢。这类梅核气疾病与心情有直接关系，对于身体疾病合并心理因素的患者，我想起以往产后抑郁的病患，心理支持和干预能使治疗事半功倍。"

传统病历是以重点记录疾病诊断、诊疗为主的记录资料，而叙事医学的要求应增加关于患者心理层面的疾苦、患者及家属的顾虑以及医务人员观察反应的医患互动记录，可以体现医务人员、患者及家属的心理与实践活动。引入"平行病历"，也正是让医师在书写标准的临床病历之外，还要用非技术性语言书写患者的体验和感受。叙事医学中的平行病历不是要把医师培养成"作者"，而是培养成更好的"医师"。

医学不完美，医师、患者有欠缺，需要包容、需要沟通、需要彼此之间的倾听。医学技术再发达也不是万能的，医者需要了解患者在疾病之外的生命境况，与患者同呼吸、共患难，达到共情、共识。平行病历的书写不分医师的年龄、年资、科室，即使是刚进入临床的住院医师，只要有一颗善感的心、一支勤奋的笔，就能把自己投入到患者的真实痛苦中去，就能写出对疾病不一样的感悟。

平行病历书写能力不佳的医师，根据教科书上的诊疗规范治疗疾病，虽然也可以积累一定的经验，但总会觉得自己与患者之间隔着一堵墙，这个隔阂无论怎么努力都无法逾越，怎么悉心照顾都仿佛缺少真情实感。而用心的书写平行病历,就会使医者豁然开悟,撕开这层与患者心中的隔膜。

六、课后习题

以叙事医学形式书写一个你感触较深的病例,要求在 300 字以上。

参考文献

[1] 卡伦.叙事医学:尊重疾病的故事[M].郭莉萍,译.北京:北京大学医学出版社,2015.

[2] 邓蕊,梁辰.医学伦理学视角下探讨叙事医学的平行病历[J].医学与哲学,2018,39(7B).13－16.

[3] 杨秋莉,王永炎.叙事医学的平行病历与中医学的医案医话[J].现代中医临床,2015,22(3).1－4.

Chapter Eight

TCM Parallel Case Writing Method

Medical record is the record of a series of medical activities for each patient from the occurrence, development, outcome, auxiliary examination, diagnosis, treatment plan and so on. Disease and suffering are two different worlds. The former is the world of medical staff, the latter is the world of patients. In the process of diagnosis and treatment, medical staff focuses on treating, observing and recording diseases, while patients experience and narrate suffering. Medical staff is in the objective world of searching for causes and pathological indicators, while patients are in the subjective world of complaining of physical and mental pain.

Modern medicine can't solve all problems. Sometimes it's a cure, often a comfort. In order to shorten the distance of trust with patients, establish the love between doctors and patients, and become the community of doctors and patients' emotions, medical workers can master the method of writing parallel medical records to improve doctors' empathy ability accompanying with medical development.

1. Definition

Parallel case emphasizes on the records of patients' subjective pain and experiences, and it is a way to introduce the idea of narrative medicine to clinic. Narrative medicine advocates that through the training of clinicians' narrative ability of understanding, interpretation and feedback, thus improving their understanding, empathy and affinity ability to their patients, and to promote the introspection of their own medical behavior.

The traditional medical records described above chapters is a kind of formatted medical records, actually in regards to traditional medical records and parallel medical records they are two ways of telling a story.

TCM always takes humanistic care as major consideration, and medical records are the specific performance and important carrier of narrative medicine's connotation in TCM. Under the background of paying attention to humanistic care and patients' subjective experience, the exploration of TCM's advantages and the construction of TCM's parallel case contain significant theoretical meaning and clinical value.

The "five faults" discussed in "Suwen Shuwuguoluan" refers to the five kinds of faults that are easily committed by doctors in the diagnosis and treatment of diseases, including neglecting the changes of patients' social status, changes of their thoughts and emotions, the state of internal mental injury, the course of illness and the principle of unknown pulse diagnosis. The five kinds of faults that occur in misdiagnosis and mistreatment clarify the psychological and social pathogenic factors and emphasize the etiology and pathogenesis of "illness is endogenous" and "psychosomatic integration". This situation is more easily understood in the form of parallel medical records.

Parallel medical records require medical students or young doctors to prepare two medical records for the same patient in clinic: one is a standard clinical medical record which is described objectively physiological and pathological indications. Doctors are looking for the objective world of etiology and pathological indicators, which are observed and recorded. The other is the parallel medical record, which is written by the doctor. It is the patient's story and his own humanistic observation and reaction. It is a subjective and narrated story of personality and humanity which is hidden in the patient's pain story, including the social and psychological roles represented by the disease, the symbolic significance, the emotional changes and the concepts and beliefs implied by the disease.

2. Differences between Parallel Medical Records and Formatted Medical Records

Traditional formatted medical records have certain layout, the order cannot be reversed. It is based on the objective description, cannot be extended from the symptom, cannot be guessed, and as long as the illness is clearly explained, reasonably introduced clinical diagnosis, the work of medical records is done. When writing a formatted medical record, the doctor is objective; he should keep calm and have a definite template, which could not be broken through at will. From the main complaint, current medical history, past history to personal history, word number, order, medical terms, or symptoms description could not be subjectively played. Parallel medical records, focusing on the doctor's concern for the patient's suffering, reproduce the patient's experience and feelings through the doctor's sympathy, and then accept the doctor into the patient's empathy circle. Both doctors and patients work to fight the disease hand in hand.

Emotional injection in parallel medical records reproduces the collision between doctors and patients, and embodies the humanistic value of medicine. Parallel medical records have no fixed pattern. In addition to basic medical skills, they need more humanistic tolerance and more emotional integration.

The purpose of parallel medical records is in line with narrative medicine. By narrating diseases, we can connect patients, diseases and suffering, connect the biological world of diseases and the life world of human beings, so that diseases can be explained and meaningful.

3. How to Write Parallel Medical Records: First Writing Diseases and Next Writing Emotions

Parallel medical records are "illness" + "emotion". It is the patient's real disease experience, both the manifestation of the disease, psychological pressure, and more confusion. In addition to the traditional medical record, it gives patients the opportunity to complain their illness, and encourages them to whisper what they want to say but are not accustomed to and dare not say. Doctors should open up their own "radar", not only to record questions, but also to listen to the patient's "illocutionary meaning", and even actively guess the patient's metaphor. Besides the rigorous format of the medical record, the doctor can't ignore the emotion. The patient's passions and desires must be as clear as his palm.

Parallel medical records talk about feelings and psychology, which requires literary connotations, philosophical thinking and reading classics particularly humanities books. Writing parallel medical records does not need to be deliberately mysterious, do not need to preach, brag, as long as it is with sincerity, even if there are no vigorous events, only with real and vivid details it can hit the hearts of the people.

What can we gain from parallel medical records Parallel medical records are also meaningful for doctors. This enables them to pay close attention to the real experience of patients in the process of diagnosis and treatment, and improve their ability to consider problems from the perspective of patients, which is also an indispensable part of medical training. And the medical record of TCM is exactly the combination of standard medical record and parallel medical record. The parallel medical records of TCM based on the medical records of TCM accord with the background and environment of attaching importance to clinical humanistic care, and which provide a scientific and effective communication platform for both doctors and patients at present.

Writing parallel medical records can improve doctors' job burnout. Because it does not have the restriction of rules, and can let you freely sprinkle feelings, with the help of a variety of stories, to let patients get rid of internal pressure and confusion.

Parallel medical records can help doctors find more clinical value than laboratory data and images, like patients' experience of disease, understanding of disease treatment and clinical medical significance. It also gives doctors more opportunities to reflect on clinical matters. Parallel medical records also allow doctors to integrate into patient's situation and to understand their feelings. This enables doctors to predict the future condition of patients to have full consideration and psychological preparations for fear of the pain and death of the disease they will face in the future.

A well-trained reader can connect with the novelist's mind, and the narrator and listener of the story can interact with each other. It is a way to restore medical humanities by letting doctors and patients collide with each other and then achieve the communication between the souls. Parallel medical records can make doctors more modest, more respectful of patients, more able to think from the standpoint of patients, and discover the further meaning of the profession of doctors.

4. Key Points of Writing Parallel Medical Records

The parallel medical records of TCM have been reflected in the medical records of ancient times. In the *Biography of Zhu Danxi*, a multipara complained of something outstanding in vulva place, like clothes. Other doctors could not find the reason. Doctor Zhu Danxi explained it was the uterus, which was caused by deficiency of Qi and Blood, so part of uterus moved out following the infant. He proscribed her Huangqi and Danggui, with Shengma to drink, and decocted Wubeizi to soak the outstanding part of her uterus. After a while her uterus raised up. At last Doctor Zhu consoled her "Three years later, you can conceive children, don't worry about it.".

This is an excerpt from the biography of celebrities, and it is not a standard medical record, but the records at that time not only clarified who was using what medicine to treat the disease, but also recorded Zhu Danxi's concern about patients' psychological comfort, "three years later, you can conceive children, don't worry about it". On the one hand, it reflects the benevolence of doctors; it also reflects that medical records attached great importance to humanistic care at that time, reflecting the interaction between doctors and patients. Case record is not just description and summary of diseases, but also shows the sincerest concern of doctors for patients and the joy and comfort of patients. Such a description method is that the parallel medical records in narrative medicine of TCM are written in a way that pays close attention to patients' feelings.

In the text of parallel medical records, we focus on a detail called close reading. In fact, when doctors write parallel medical records, they can understand the real sufferings of patients better through the writing of the text. Through careful reading of this text, we can examine our psychological changes and intervention process in clinical practice. The three important elements of parallel medical records are attention, reproduction and action. Attention is to focus on those circumstances, to reproduce the situation at that time, and to take correct and reasonable action to make the patient get a better mood and help the recovery of the disease.

5. Parallel Medical Record Format

5. 1　Definition of parallel medical records　Parallel medical records, as the writing format of narrative medicine, are mainly composed of five parts, which include time、plot、imagine、empathy (feeling/emotion) and significance.

5. 2　Examples of parallel medical records of TCM　Through the study of ancient books of TCM and clinical practice of personal participation, a parallel medical record of TCM was written down.

On the autumn equinox of September 15, 2014, a 45-year-old middle-aged woman came to the clinic with gaunt complexion and a feeling of foreign body obstructing in her chest for two months. All kinds of examinations were unsuccessful. She cried and lost her voice when describing her illness. She felt it was aggravating that she was not breathing well. After careful inquiring, I learned that her husband had lost his job, had been drinking at home for a long time, and did not care about her children. She had been a full-time housewife, had no financial resources, and had no ability to make a living. It was common to have quarrels at home. Later, every time she came to consult a doctor, she had to talk for a long time, including whether the child was obedient recently and how many her grades were. When she talked about the child, her eyes shone with different light, as if that was the straw in her life. The patient's tongue is dull and fur is thin, white and greasy. The diagnosis of this disease is "globus hysteriocus" in TCM. In addition to TCM therapy, psychotherapy is particularly important. The patient's conscious symptoms were relieved, and her chest was relaxed for half a year, but she did not recover. Sometimes the symptoms were aggravated repeatedly, it often related to quarrels and depression. Later, after repeated studies of her medical records and conditions, in addition to medication, guidance and other treatment, I also gave her advice on getting out of the house, into the community and participating in social work recommendations. The patient went to a local private kindergarten to help with the kitchen. On the one hand, she could relieve her depression; She could also ease the financial burden of her family. About three months later, the patient came to the clinic to thank me with joy. This kind of globus hysteriocus disease has a direct relationship with emotion. For patients with physical diseases and psychological factors, I think of patients with postpartum depression in the past. Psychological support and intervention can often make the treatment more effective.

Traditional medical records mainly record the diagnosis and treatment of diseases. Narrative medicine requires that more records of patients' psychological distress, the concerns of patients and their families, and the doctor-patient interaction of medical staff's observation and response should be added to reflect the psychological and practical activities of medical staff, patients and their families. The introduction of "parallel medical records" is not only to enable doctors to write standard clinical records, but also to use non-technical language to write patients' experience and feelings. Parallel medical records in narrative medicine do not train doctors to be "authors", but to be better "doctors".

Medical science is not perfect. Doctors and patients are deficient. They need tolerance, communication and listening to each other. The development of medical technology is not omnipotent. Doctors need to know about patients' lives outside the disease, breathe and suffer with patients, and reach sympathy and consensus. Parallel medical records are written regardless of the age, seniority and department of the doctor. Even the resident who has just entered the clinic can put himself into the real pain of the patient as long as he has a sympathetic heart and a diligent pen.

Doctors with poor parallel medical record writing ability treat diseases according to the diagnostic and therapeutic criteria in textbooks. Although they can accumulate certain experience, they will feel that there is a wall between themselves and patients one day. No matter how hard you try, this gap cannot be overcome, and how carefully you take care of it seems that there is a lack of true authenticity. Writing parallel medical records attentively will make the doctor suddenly enlighten and eliminate the estrangement from the patients.

6. Homework

Write a case in the form of narrative medicine that you have a deep feeling for. It requires more than 300 words.

References

[1] Charon R. Narrative medicine: honoring the stories ofIllness [M]. New York: Oxford University Press, 2006: 155 – 174.

[2] Deng R, Liang C. Parallel medical records of narrative medicine from the perspective of medical ethics [J]. Medicine and Philosophy, 2018. 39 (7B). 13 – 16.

[3] Yang Q, Wang Y. Parallel medical records of narrative medicine and medical records of traditional Chinese medicine[J]. Modern Chinese Medicine Clinical, 2015, 22 (3). 1 – 4.

第九章

GB95 和 GB97,中国中医诊断国家标准

本章节将为您简单介绍关于中医病证分类与代码(简称"95 国标",GB95)和中医临床诊疗术语(简称"97 国标",GB97)的定义以及编码方法。

一、定义

若有机会观察中国公立医疗机构——医院或诊所中的中医病案,您可以很容易地找到标准化的中医诊断编码。事实上,自 1995 年以来,病和证相关的国标(GB)就已正式发布:GB95 和发布于 1997 年的 GB97 并称为中医标准化的里程碑。随着它们的实施,我们收集并分析了越来越多来自不同级别医疗机构记录患者的中医数据。标准化代码使我们能够比较中国不同地区的数据,或者更准确地在国家层面进行计算。这两部国标帮助政府和中医从业人员推动了医疗服务、培训、科学研究、临床试验、卫生统计、出版物和相关政策等工作的进步。

二、编码方法

通常,在 TCM 实践中用于编码诊断的代码来自 GB95。不幸的是,在 GB95 中,您只能找到相关代码的中医疾病和模式的分类,但没有定义。在 GB97 中,每个 TCM 术语实体都遵循一个简短的定义。

在 GB95 中,中医诊断分为两类:中医病(疾病)和中医证(证候)。

1. 中医病(疾病)编码规则　中医病的实体分为 7 类,包括:内科疾病,外科疾病,妇科疾病,儿科疾病,眼科疾病,耳鼻喉科疾病和骨科疾病。典型中医病实体的代码通常包含 6 位编码。病的编码规则如下(图 9-1)。

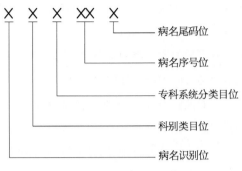

图 9-1 中医病（疾病）编码规则

病名标识位：B，取病的第一个拼音字母，汉语拼音 Bing。

科别类目位：取每个子类的汉语拼音的第一个字母。

专科系统分类目位：取每个临床科室的汉语拼音的第一个字母。

病名序号位：在每个类别相关的病类目下，每个病实体都分配了唯一的编码。

病名尾码位：当病需要进一步分类时，该数字将是标签，并以阿拉伯数字标明。

例如：BNX070 癫狂、BNX071 癫病、BNX072 狂病。

B，Bing 的第一个字母，"病"。

N，内科（Neike）的第一个字母，"内科"。

X，心系病的第一个字母（Xinxibing Lei），"心系病类"。

07，这些实体的病名序号。

0，1，2 是这些实体的尾码。

2. **中医证（证候）编码规则** 中医证候实体分为 6 个亚类，包括：病因证候，阴阳、气血、津液、痰证候，脏腑、经络证候，六经证候，卫气营血证候，其他证候（图 9-2）。

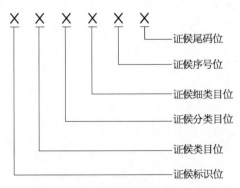

图 9-2 证候编码规则

证候识别位：Z，取证汉语拼音的第一个字母，汉语拼音"Zheng"。

证的序号位：取中文音译类的第一个字母。

证候分类目位：取每个分类的中文音译的第一个字母。

证候细类目位：取每个细类目的中文音译的第一个字母。

证候序号位：在每个类别的证候中，每个证候实体都分配了一个唯一的编码，以阿拉伯数字（0~9）标准，在必要时续用字母 A~Z 标记。

证候尾码位：当证候需要进一步分类时，该码位为标签，以阿拉伯数字标记。

例如：ZBF010 风邪袭表证；ZBF011 风邪外袭证；ZBF012 风邪外袭，经气痞塞证；ZBF013 风邪侵袭证。

Z，证的第一个字母，"Zheng"。

B，病因证候类拼音 Bingyin Zhenghou Lei 的第一个字母。

F，风证类的首字母（Fengzheng Lei）。

第一个"0"，是风证类的序号。

第一个"1"，用于风邪袭表证的序列号。

最后的 0，1，2 和 3 是尾码位。

对于从事人工编码的编码员来说，知晓上述编码规则将使这些代码更易读易懂，故而需要慎重。近年来，随着健康信息系统的发展，编码员只需记住标准化诊断，而他们的计算机将自动分配代码到诊断。除此之外，这些代码也可以用作研究病和证的层次结构，以及用作确定所分配的代码是否合适的一个线索。

Chapter Nine

International Classification of Case in TCM Medicine

This chapter will briefly introduce the definition and encoding method of Classification and Codes of Diseases and Zheng of Traditional Chinese Medicine (GB95) and Clinic Terminology of Traditional Chinese Medicine Diagnosis and Treatment(GB97).

1. Definition

If you get a chance to look at TCM records in government running medical care facilities in China, such as hospitals and clinics, you may notice the standardized codes of TCM diagnosis. As a matter of fact, since 1995, the GB(Guo Biao, National Standard) on Bing (diseases) and Zheng(patterns) has been officially released as the Classification and Codes of Diseases and Zheng of Traditional Chinese Medicine(GB95). In 1997, another GB on TCM terms has been officially released: Clinic Terminology of Traditional Chinese Medicine Diagnosis and Treatment(GB97). Those two GBs serve as milestones of TCM standardization. With their implement, more and more TCM data from patient records in different level of health care facilities can be collected and analyzed. The standardized codes allow us to compare data from different regions of China and study them at a national level more easily and precisely. The two GBs have helped practitioners and government improve medical care, training, scientific research, clinical trial, health statistics, publications and related policies, etc.

2. Encoding Method

Generally, the codes which are used to code diagnosis in TCM practice are from GB95. Unfortunately, in GB95 only gives the classification of TCM diseases and patterns with related codes, but no definition. In contrast, GB97 includes a short definition for, each entity of TCM terms.

In GB95, TCM diagnosis were sorted into two categories: TCM Bing(diseases) and Zheng (patterns).

2.1 The coding rules of TCM Bing (diseases) The entities of TCM Bing were classified into 7 sub-classes, including: diseases of internal medicine, surgery, gynecology, paediatrics, ophthalmology, ENT (ear, nose and throat) and orthopedics. The code for a typical Bing entity usually contents 6 digits. The coding rules of Bing were as Figure 9 – 1.

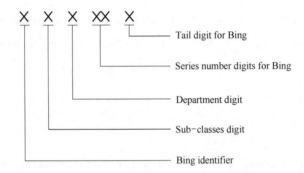

Figure 9 – 1 The coding rules of TCM Bing (diseases)

Bing identifier: B, take the first letter of Bing, the Chinese transliteration of character "病".

Sub-classes digit: take the first letter from the Chinese transliteration of each sub-classes.

Department digit: take the first letter from the Chinese transliteration of each clinical departments.

Series number digits for Bing: under each category of department related Bing, each entity of Bing was allotted with a unique code.

Tail digit: when a Bing needs to be classified furtherly, this digit would be the label, and labelled with Arabic number.

E.g.:

BNX070 癫狂病　　Depressive and manic psychosis.

BNX071 癫病　　　Depressive psychosis.

BNX072 狂病　　　Manic psychosis.

B, the first letter of Bing, 病.

N, the first letter of Neike(internal medicine), 内科.

X, the first letter of Xinxibing Lei(Category of heart system diseases),心系病类.

07, the series number digits of this entity.

0,1,2 are the tail digits of those entities.

2.2 The entities of TCM Zheng were classified into 6 subclasses The 6 subclasses includ etiological patterns, patterns of Yin, Yang, Qi, blood, body fluid and phlegm, six stage patterns, patterns of defense Qi, nutrient and blood aspects.

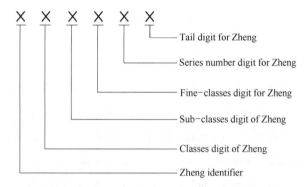

Figure 9 - 2 The coding rules of TCM Zheng (pattens)

Zheng identifier: Z, take the first letter of Zheng, the Chinese transliteration of character "Zheng".

Classes digit of Zheng: take the first letter from the Chinese transliteration of classes.

Sub-classes digit: take the first letter from the Chinese transliteration of each subclasses.

Fine-classes digit: take the first letter from the Chinese transliteration of each fine-classes.

Series number digit for Zheng: under each category of department related Zheng, each entity of Zheng was allotted with a unique code, labelled with Arabic number (0 - 9), then letter A - Z if necessary.

Tail digit: when a Zheng needs to be classified furtherly, this digit would be the label, and labelled with Arabic number.

E.g.:

ZBF010 Pattern of pathogenic wind assailing the exterior 风邪袭表证

ZBF011 Pattern of exterior assailing of pathogenic wind 风邪外袭证

ZBF012 Pattern of pathogenic wind assailing the exterior with meridian Qi block 风邪外袭, 经气痹塞证

ZBF013 Pattern of pathogenic wind intruding and assailing 风邪侵袭证

Z, the first letter of Zheng(pattern), 证.

B, the first letter of Bingyin Zhenghou Lei (category of etiological patterns), 病因证候类.

F, the first letter of Feng Zheng Lei(Category of wind patterns), 风证类.

The first "0", the series number of pathogenic wind patterns.

The first "1", the series number for the patterns of pathogenic wind assailing the exterior.

The last "0", "1", "2" and "3" are tail digits.

Understanding the principles behind the coding rules above will make the codes more readable and understandable. It is very important for coders to manually allot codes to diagnosis. In recent years, with the development of health informatics systems, all the coders need to do is to remember the standardized diagnosis, while their computers will allot codes to the diagnosis automatically. However, the codes can also be used as a clue for studying the hierarchy of disorders and patterns and a way to determine whether the allotted codes are appropriate.

第十章　中医疾病编码与应用

本章分为以下几个部分：定义，国际疾病分类史，ICD－10、ICD－11 和中国的双重编码系统，如何在线检索 ICD 诊断编码（以 ICD－11 为例），国际疾病分类的功能，如何以简单的方式更好地利用复杂的编码系统，阅读材料和课后习题。

一、定义

诊断是医疗记录中最重要的部分之一。我们从问诊、查体、实验室检查、放射成像和形态学中获得的所有信息都经过仔细分析和总结，以支持最终诊断。如今，诊断不仅用于医疗保健，为每个诊断分配标准化代码有助于我们从计算机系统轻松提取数据。这些数据将有助于我们改善医疗保健，起草疾病管理战略和指导方针，支持政府的卫生政策，当然还有助于科学研究。疾病最重要的国际编码系统之一是国际疾病分类（ICD），用于表示国际疾病和相关疾病分类。它是世界卫生组织（WHO）的标准化计数工具。我们使用的最新版本是 ICD－10。到目前为止，已有 130 多个国家使用这种编码系统。

ICD 由 WHO 维护，WHO 是联合国系统内健康的指导和协调机构。ICD 被设计为医疗保健分类系统，提供疾病分类诊断代码系统，包括细致的分类，各种各样的体征、症状、异常发现、主诉、社会环境因素以及导致受伤或疾病的外因。该系统旨在将健康状况与特定变量一起映射到相应的通用类别，并为其分配长达六位的代码。因此，主要类别被设计为包括一组类似的疾病。

ICD 由 WHO 出版，在世界范围内用于发病率和死亡率统计，报销系统以及医疗保健中的自动决策支持。该系统旨在促进这些数据的收集、处理、分类和表示方面的国际可比性。与类似的精神疾病诊断和统计手册（仅限于精神疾病）一样，ICD 是对所有健康、疾病进行统计分类并提供诊断帮助的主要分类。它是世界卫生组织国际分类家族（WHO－FIC）卫生保健相关问题的核心统计分类诊断系统。

ICD 定期修订，其最新正式发布的版本为 ICD‐10。自 1992 年以来，WHO 每年都会发布一些小的更新和 3 年一次的主要更新。ICD 第 11 次修订的项目于 2010 年启动。ICD‐11 原计划于 2017 年正式发布，但由于不明原因，它被推迟到 2019 年。作为 WHO‐FIC 家族的重要组成部分，ICD 有两个姐妹分类。它们是 ICF（国际功能，残疾和健康分类）和 ICHI（国际健康干预分类）。从医学和社会角度来看，ICF 主要关注与健康状况相关的功能（残疾）领域。ICHI 涵盖了整个卫生系统范围的广泛提供者的干预措施，包括如下：诊断、医疗、外科、心理健康、初级保健、专职医疗、功能支持、康复、传统医学和公共卫生。

二、国际疾病分类史

1860 年，在伦敦举行的国际统计大会期间，弗洛伦斯·南丁格尔提出了关于开发第一个系统收集医院数据模型的建议。1891 年，国际统计学会指定由雅克·波提顿博士（1851—1922）领导的一个委员会，对死因进行分类。该草案于 1893 年在芝加哥会议期间获得通过。1898 年，美国公共卫生协会建议采用波提顿在美国的分类。

1900 年，法国政府召开了第一次修订波提顿/或国际死亡原因分类国际会议。来自 26 个国家的代表出席了会议。所采用的分类有 179 种死亡原因，还通过了包涵 35 种死因类别的简化版本。这是 ICD 的第一次修订，是自 1955 年以来应用于该系列的雏形，尽管标题略有修改且内容范围不断扩大。1946 年，联合国将 ICD 修订的责任移交给 WHO，后者拟定了第六版和随后的修订版本。ICD‐6（1948 年）列入了发病率和死亡率统计的综合列表，有助于在全世界建立国家卫生和人口动态统计委员会，并加强卫生统计活动的国际协调。第四十三届世界卫生大会于 1990 年 5 月批准了 ICD‐10。到目前为止，ICD‐10 是最新和最广泛采用的版本，已用于临床数据收集和科学研究。

ICD 是目前世界上使用最广泛的疾病统计分类系统。此外，许多国家，如澳大利亚、加拿大和美国，已经开发了自己的 ICD 修订本，纳入更多的手术操作代码用于操作或诊断干预的分类。

通常 ICD 的国家修订本包括更多细节编码，有时还有单独的手术操作分类。例如，美国 ICD‐10 临床修改（ICD‐10‐CM）有大约 68 000 个代码。美国也有 ICD‐10 程序编码系统（ICD‐10‐PCS），一个包含 76 000 个并未在其他国家或地区使用的手术操作编码系统。

三、ICD‐10、ICD‐11 和中国的双重编码系统

1. ICD‐10　ICD‐10 是 WHO 的医学分类列表 ICD 的第十版。它包含疾病、体征和症

状,异常发现、主诉、社会环境因素以及导致受伤或疾病的外部原因的代码。

代码集纳入超过 14 400 种不同的代码,并允许统计许多新的诊断。通过使用可选的子分类,代码数量可以扩展到超过 16 000 个。

WHO 在线提供有关 ICD 的详细信息,并在线提供一套资料,如 ICD‐10 在线浏览器,ICD‐10 培训,ICD‐10 在线培训,ICD‐10 在线培训支持材料和学习指南材料下载。

关于 ICD‐10 的修订工作始于 1983 年,并于 1992 年完成。通过以下链接,使用百度或谷歌等搜索工具,您可以轻松访问官方网站(图 10‐1):http://apps.who.int/classifications/icd10/browse/2010/en。

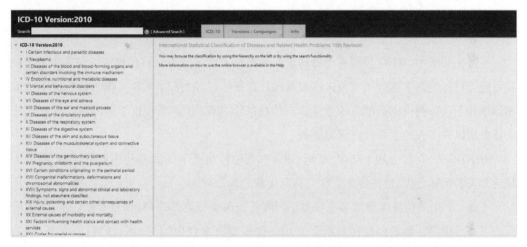

图 10‐1 ICD‐10 浏览器的用户界面(UI)

在该用户界面的左侧是整个 ICD‐10 的框架。当您选择左侧的某些项目时,详细的代码和信息将显示在右侧(图 10‐2)。

但是,在 ICD‐10 中,除了层次结构和编码之外,您几乎找不到每个概念的详细定义。

2. ICD‐11(冻结版) WHO 目前正在修订 ICD 的第十一版国际疾病分类 ICD‐11。编写工作是在基于互联网的系统上进行的,该系统称为 iCAT(协作编辑工具)平台。WHO 组织了所有相关领域的专家,为 ICD‐11 的修订做出贡献。

ICD‐11 最终草案于 2019 年提交 WHO 世界卫生大会(WHA)正式批准。同行评审已于 2018 年完成,冻结版现可在线获取。它被宣布为最终版本,在 2019 年 WHA 期间获得批准并正式发布。

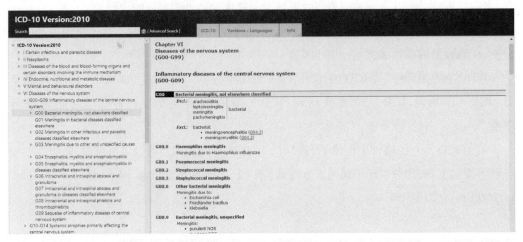

图 10 - 2　详细代码和信息

在过去几年中，WHO 为促进全球传统医学做出了巨大努力。将传统医学纳入 ICD‐11 有可能为将传统医学整合入主流医疗记录和计费系统打开大门。ICD‐11 为传统医学术语和诊断和干预分类提供标准化的数据库。传统医学是亚洲、非洲和拉丁美洲以及欧洲和北美部分地区许多人的主要医疗保健资源。

WHO 认为，在过去几十年中，草药、针灸和其他传统医学实践的使用显著增加，但由于缺乏相关的国际分类，这些数据无法在国际上收集和比较。

ICD‐11 中的传统医学章节主要基于国际传统医学分类(ICTM)项目专家的工作，他们代表了来自世界各地的广泛传统医学知识。许多专家来自中国、日本、韩国、澳大利亚、美国、英国、荷兰和其他一些国家。

参与同行评审的专家也可以提出修订 ICD‐11 的建议，以解决缺失的内容，或根据新的理解和信息提供更新。通过这一过程，WHO 打算利用具有医疗保健专业知识的最广泛的个人群体来确保尽可能准确以及最新的信息。

形成国际传统医学分类的潜在好处包括：① 将传统医学实践与全球规范和标准制订联系起来。② 加强全球统计，监测公共安全方面的国际公共卫生任务。③ 支持世界各地传统医学从实验室到临床的研究。④ 帮助所有 WHO 193 个成员国平等获取全球公共产品。⑤ 将传统医学纳入全球统计。⑥ 促进中医保健医保报销。

总而言之，此版本中有几个新功能。此外，代码和层次结构，每个概念都有一个简短的定义。已经设计了基于本体的内容模型，专家可以用这些模型定义每个概念。在这种情况下，在不久的将来，计算机系统将全面理解所有代码、定义、分类和层次结构。通过这种智能网络，专家可以轻松获取数据并充分利用它们。

ICD-11最重要的新功能之一是传统医学(TM)章节。它是传统医学的独立篇章。在这个阶段,TM指的是中医。未来,更多的传统药物将加入ICD家庭。由于章节空间有限,ICD-11的TM章节中只包含有限的实体。但是整个中医诊断框架已经引入本章。希望在不久的将来,TCM诊断的整个价值将在ICTM项目的专著中提供。

通过以下链接,您可以轻松访问ICD-11 Beta浏览器(图10-3):http://apps.who.int/classifications/icd11/browse/f/en。

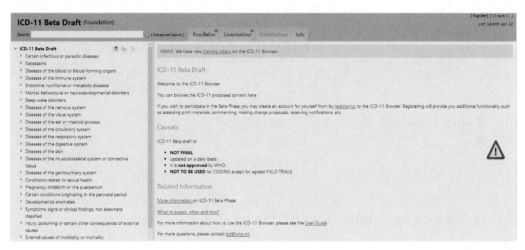

图10-3 ICD-11 Beta浏览器

3. 中国双编码系统 目前在中国,在中医医院和中医相关科室,正在使用一种称为双编码系统的编码系统。在这个系统中,医师使用ICD-10代码编码大多数是所谓的西医诊断,ICD-9 CM3编码手术操作,以及用TCD编码中医诊断。TCD码也称为GB代码。GB95主要是关于中医诊断的分类和编码,包括疾病和证候。GB97主要涉及临床术语。当我们进行中医诊断时,有两个必要的部分。一部分是疾病或疾患编码,另一部分是证候代码。这两个标准的官方修订版处于同行审查阶段。据悉两国标的新版本将于近期发布并实施。

四、如何在线检索ICD诊断编码(以ICD-11为例)

1. 病案 某60岁女性患者,3个月前被诊断为糖尿病,患者口渴,多尿,多饮,口干咽燥,急躁易怒,盗汗。舌质红少津,苔薄黄,脉弦。

2. 检索操作

（1）打开网络搜索引擎。以百度（www.baidu.com）为例，如图 10-4 所示。

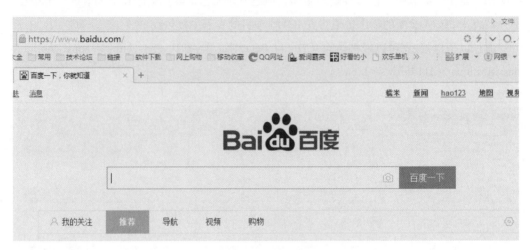

图 10-4　百度搜索页面

（2）在搜索栏中输入"ICD-11 WHO"，如图 10-5 所示。

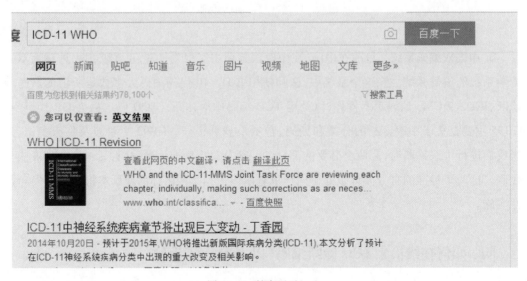

图 10-5　搜索页面（一）

（3）点击"WHO│ICD-11 Revision"，如图10-6所示。

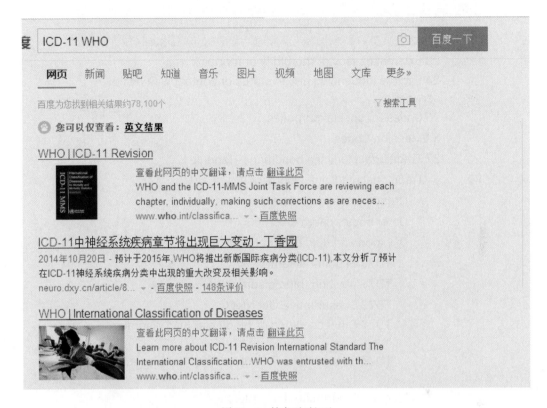

图10-6 搜索页面(二)

4）搜索中医无序代码，如图10-7所示。① 首先点击"27章传统医学—模块Ⅰ"。② 第二步"气，血液和津液病（TM）"。③ 第三次点击"TD71 消渴病（TM）"。

结果：中医病证编号为TD71。

5）搜索TCM的证候编码，如图10-8所示。① 首先点击"传统医学证候（TM）"。② 第二次点击"肺系证候（TM）"。③ 第三次点击"TF72 肺阴虚证（TM）"。

结果：中医证候编码为TF72。

6）检索西医疾病代码，如图10-9所示。

✓ ICD-11 Beta Draft - Mortality and M ↻

▶ 23 External causes of morbidity or mortality

▶ 24 Factors influencing health status or contact with health services

▶ 25 Codes for special purposes

▶ X Extension Codes

▽ 27 Traditional Medicine conditions - Module I

    ▽ Traditional medicine disorders (TM)

        ▶ Organ system disorders (TM)

        ▶ Other body system disorders (TM)

        ▽ Qi, blood and fluid disorders (TM)   83%

            TD70 Qi goiter disorder (TM)

            TD71 Wasting thirst disorder (TM)

            TD72 Consumptive disorder (TM)

            TD7Y Other specified qi, blood and fluid disorders (TM)

            TD7Z Qi, blood and fluid disorders (TM) , unspecified

        ▶ Mental and emotional disorders (TM)

        ▶ External contraction disorders (TM)

        ▶ Childhood and adolescence associated disorders (TM)

        TE5Y Other specified traditional medicine disorders (TM)

        TE5Z Traditional medicine disorders (TM) , unspecified

    ▶ Traditional medicine patterns (TM)

    TJ2Y Other specified traditional Medicine conditions - Module I

    TJ2Z Traditional Medicine conditions - Module I, unspecified

图 10 - 7　搜索中医无序代码

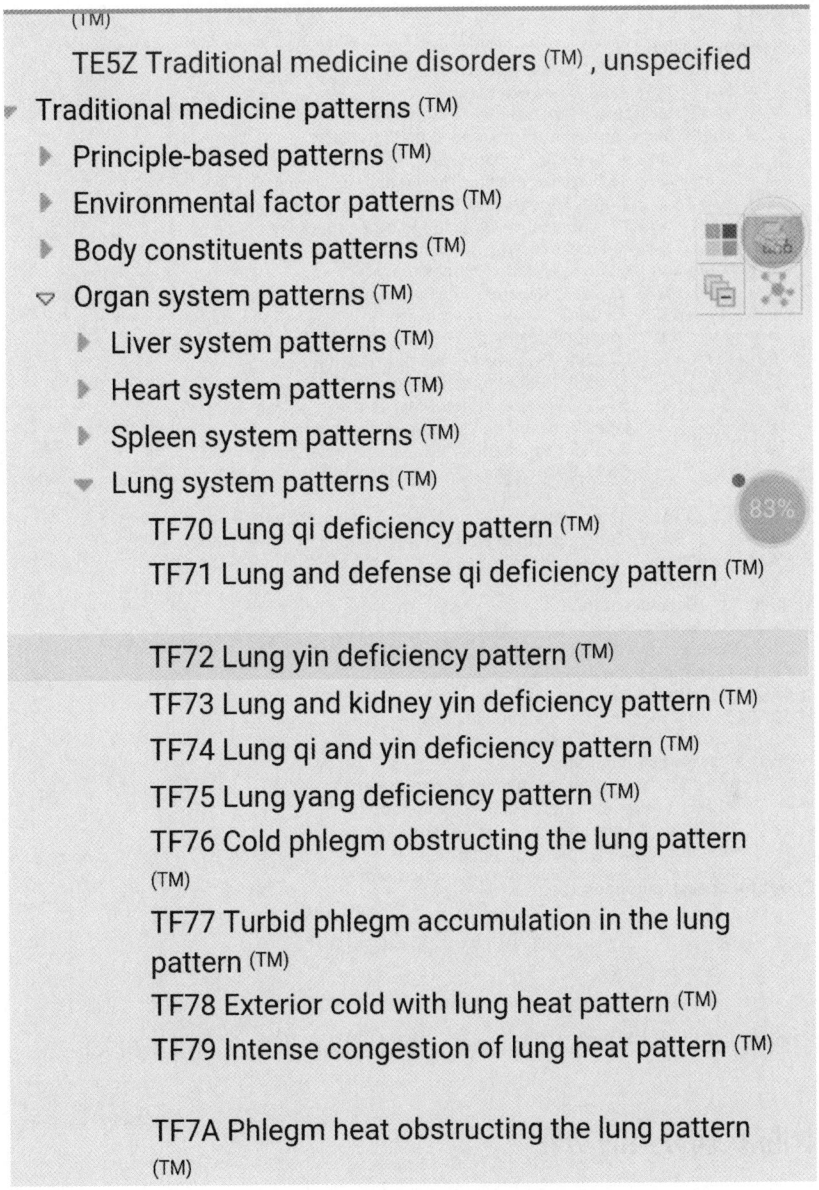

(TM)

TE5Z Traditional medicine disorders (TM) , unspecified

▾ Traditional medicine patterns (TM)

▸ Principle-based patterns (TM)

▸ Environmental factor patterns (TM)

▸ Body constituents patterns (TM)

▽ Organ system patterns (TM)

  ▸ Liver system patterns (TM)

  ▸ Heart system patterns (TM)

  ▸ Spleen system patterns (TM)

  ▾ Lung system patterns (TM)

TF70 Lung qi deficiency pattern (TM)

TF71 Lung and defense qi deficiency pattern (TM)

TF72 Lung yin deficiency pattern (TM)

TF73 Lung and kidney yin deficiency pattern (TM)

TF74 Lung qi and yin deficiency pattern (TM)

TF75 Lung yang deficiency pattern (TM)

TF76 Cold phlegm obstructing the lung pattern (TM)

TF77 Turbid phlegm accumulation in the lung pattern (TM)

TF78 Exterior cold with lung heat pattern (TM)

TF79 Intense congestion of lung heat pattern (TM)

TF7A Phlegm heat obstructing the lung pattern (TM)

图 10 - 8　搜索 TCM 的证候编码

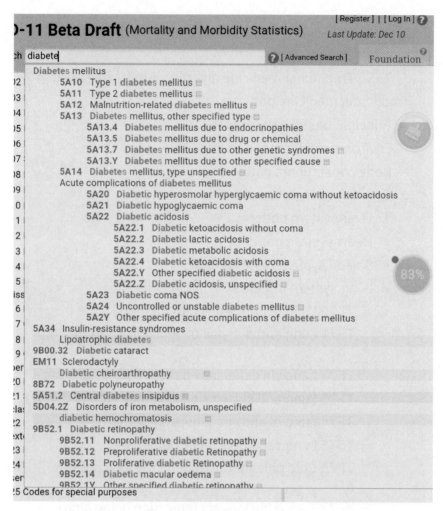

图 10-9 检索西医疾病代码

根据本病案,在搜索栏中输入"diabete",我们可以在下面看到很多相关信息。

五、国际疾病分类的功能

当我们从不同的国家或地区收集数据时,如果标准不同,我们不能将数据汇总或相互比较。如果使用相同的标准,数据的比较和分析可能会更容易。也就是说,ICD 具有统一、标准化、国际化和便利的特点。

在当前以信息为基础的社会中,ICD 加快了录入和检索的速度,这可以显著提高医务工作者的工作效率。此外,它在病历管理和临床科学研究中具有积极意义。ICD 还可以促进医疗保健提供者与来自不同国家和不同领域的国际间的交流,为世界医学发展做出巨大贡献。

六、如何更好地利用复杂的编码系统

作为医学实习生,学习一些国家和国际诊断分类知识将为您未来的工作奠定良好的基础。由于采用了计算机技术,我们不必记住复杂的代码或在一堆厚厚的书中查找它们。我们要做的所有事情,就是学习标准化诊断,熟悉它们并在日常实践中使用它们。计算机系统将帮助我们自动为每个诊断分配标准化代码。熟悉 ICD 及其浏览器数据库将使您的编码工作更加轻松高效。

七、阅读材料

(1) http：//www.who.int/classifications/icd/en/.。
(2) ICD-10 第二版第二卷。
(3) ICD 发展历史。

八、课后习题

某 37 岁男性患有胃炎,有上腹部钝痛,胸闷,口干,不欲饮,口中有黏腻,恶心,偶有呕吐。舌红,苔黄腻,脉滑数。
请检索其中医疾病和证候编码,以及西方疾病编码。

参考文献

[1] 世界卫生组织. 国际疾病分类（ICD）［EB/OL］. ［2014 - 02 - 12］. https：//www.who.int/classifications/icd/en/.

[2] 世界卫生组织. 关于 WHO［EB/OL］. (2014 - 03 - 14)［2014 - 02 - 09］.https：//www.who.int/about/en/.

[3] 世界卫生组织. WHO 中国际疾病分类［EB/OL］. (2014 - 03 - 14)［2013 - 12 - 22］. https：//www.who.int/classifications/en/.

[4] 世界卫生组织. ICD - 11 2017 年修订版［EB/OL］. ［2014 - 02 - 17］. http：//www.who.int/classifications/icd/revision/en/.

［ 5 ］世界卫生组织. ICD 发展史［EB/OL］.［2020 - 10 - 21］. https：//www.who.int/classifications/icd/en/HistoryOfICD.pdf.

［ 6 ］世界卫生组织. 国际卫生统计资料可查阅 WHO 统计信息系统数据库［EB/OL］.［2020 - 11 - 15］. https：//www.who.int/whosis/en/.

［ 7 ］世界卫生组织. 国际卫生统计资料可查阅全球卫生观察数据库［EB/OL］.［2020 - 11 - 17］. https：//www.who.int/data/gho/.

［ 8 ］疾病防治中心. ICD - 10 临床修改版：第 10 版［EB/OL］.［2015 - 12 - 02］. https：//www.cdc.gov/nchs/icd/icd10cm.htm.

［ 9 ］美国卫生与公共服务部. ICD - 10 程序编码系统及更新［EB/OL］.［2008 - 10 - 22］. https：//en.wikipedia.org/wiki/U.S._Department_of_Health_&_Human_Services.

［10］世界卫生组织. 国际疾病分类（ICD）［EB/OL］.［2010 - 11 - 23］. https：//www.who.int/classifications/icd/en/.

［11］ICD - 10. ICD - 10 官网［EB/OL］.［2015 - 12 - 20］. https：//icd.who.int/browse10/2015/en.

［12］世界卫生组织. ICD - 10 练习工具［EB/OL］.［2010 - 12 - 25］. https：//apps.who.int/classifications/apps/icd/icd10training/.

［13］ICD - 10. ICD - 10 线上支持［EB/OL］.［2015 - 12 - 23］. https：//sites.google.com/site/icd10onlinetraining.

Chapter Ten

Disease Coding and Application in TCM

This chapter is divided into following sections: definition, the history of international classification of diseases, ICD − 10 and ICD − 11 and double coding system in China, how to retrieve diagnosis in ICD online (take ICD − 11 as example), the function of ICD, how to make better use of the complicated coding system in a simple way, suggesting reading after class and homework.

1. Definition

Diagnosis is one of the most important part of medical records. All the information one obtains from inquiry, examination, laboratory tests, radiology imaging and morphology are carefully analyzed and summarized to support the final diagnosis. Nowadays, diagnosis is not only used for medical care but also to help in medical health management. To assign a standardized code for each diagnosis would help us to extract data easily from computer systems. This data would help us in improving medical care, drafting strategies and guidelines for the management of diseases, supporting health policy from governments and of course facilitating scientific research. One of the most important international coding systems for diseases is ICD, the International Classification of Diseases and Related Conditions. This is a standardized tool from World Health Organization (WHO). The latest version we're using is ICD − 10. So far, more than 130 countries are using this coding system.

ICD is maintained by WHO, the directing and coordinating authority for health within the United Nations System. ICD is designed as a health care classification system, providing a system of diagnostic codes for classifying diseases, including nuanced classifications of a wide variety of signs, symptoms, abnormal findings, complaints, social circumstances, and external causes of injury or disease. This system is designed to map health conditions to corresponding generic categories together with specific variations, assigning them with a designated code, up to six digits long. Thus, major categories are designed to include a set of similar diseases.

ICD is published by the WHO and used worldwide for morbidity and mortality statistics, reimbursement systems, and automated decision support in health care. This system is designed to promote international comparability in the collection, processing, classification, and presentation of these data. Like the analogous Diagnostic and Statistical Manual of Mental Disorders (which is limited to psychiatric disorders), ICD is a major project to statistically classify all health disorders, and provide diagnostic assistance. It is a core statistically based classificatory diagnostic system for health care related issues of the WHO Family of International Classifications (WHO – FIC).

ICD is revised periodically and its latest officially released version is ICD – 10. Since 1992, WHO has published annual minor updates and triennial major updates. The project for the 11th revision of ICD was launched in 2010. And ICD – 11 was planned to be officially released in 2017, but due to unknown reasons, it was postponed to 2019. As an important part of WHO – FIC family, ICD has two sister classifications. They are ICF (International Classification of Functioning, Disability and Health) and ICHI (International Classification of Health Interventions). ICF focuses mainly on the domains of functioning (disability) associated with health conditions, from both medical and social perspectives. ICHI covers interventions carried out by a broad range of providers across the full scope of health systems and includes interventions on: diagnostic, medical, surgical, mental health, primary care, allied health, functioning support, rehabilitation, traditional medicine and public health.

2. The History of International Classification of Diseases

In 1860, during the international statistical congress held in London, Florence Nightingale made a proposal on the development of the first model of systemic collection of hospital data. In 1891, the International Statistical Institute charged a committee headed by Dr. Jacques Bertillon (1851 – 1922) to produce a classification on causes of death. The draft was approved in 1893 during the meeting in Chicago. In 1898, the American Public Health Association recommended the adoption of Bertillon's classification in United States.

In 1900, the French government convened the first International Conference for the Revision of the Bertillon or International Classification of Causes of Death. Delegates from twenty-six countries attended the conference. The classification that was adopted had 179 categories of causes of death and an abridged version of thirty-five categories was also proved. This was the first revision of ICD, the prototype that has been applied to the series since 1955 despite slightly modified titles and expanding scope of content. In 1946, the United Nations handed over the responsibility for ICD revision to WHO, which issued the sixth and other succeeding revisions. ICD − 6 (1948) included a comprehensive list for morbidity as well as mortality statistics, which facilitated the establishment of national committees on health and vital statistics throughout the world and increased international coordination of health statistical activities. ICD − 10 was endorsed in May 1990 by the Forty-third World Health Assembly. So far, ICD − 10 is the latest and most widely adopted version which has been used for clinical data collection and scientific study.

ICD is currently the most widely used statistical classification system for diseases in the world. In addition, many countries such as Australia, Canada, and the United States — have developed their own adaptations of ICD, with more procedure codes for classification of operative or diagnostic interventions.

Usually the national modifications of ICD include more detail, and sometimes have separate sections for procedures. The US ICD − 10 Clinical Modification (ICD − 10 − CM), for instance, has about 68,000 codes. The US also has the ICD − 10 Procedure Coding System (ICD − 10 − PCS), a coding system that contains 76,000 procedure codes that is not used by other countries.

3. ICD − 10, ICD − 11 and Double Coding System in China

3.1 ICD − 10 ICD − 10 is the 10th revision of the International Statistical Classification of Diseases and Related Health Problems (ICD), a medical classification list by the WHO. It contains codes for diseases, signs and symptoms, abnormal findings, complaints, social circumstances, and external causes of injury or diseases.

The code set allows more than 14,400 different codes and permits the tracking of many new diagnoses. The codes can be expanded to over 16,000 codes by using optional sub-classifications.

The WHO provides detailed information about ICD online, and makes available a set of materials online, such as an ICD‑10 online browser, ICD‑10 training, ICD‑10 online training, ICD‑10 online training support, and study guiding materials for download.

Work on ICD‑10 revision began in 1983 and was completed in 1992.

With the link below, or with some searching tools, such as Baidu or Google, you can easily access the official website. http://apps.who.int/classifications/icd10/browse/2010/en (Figure 10‑1).

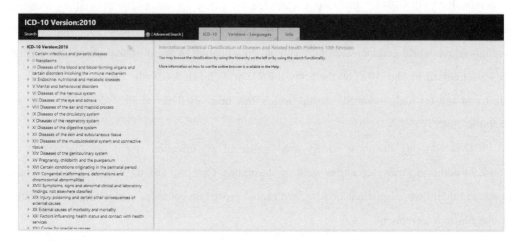

Figure 10‑1　The user interface (UI) of ICD‑10 browser.

On the left side of this UI, it is the framework of the whole ICD‑10. When you choose some specified items on the left, the detailed codes and information will be shown on the right (Figure 10‑2).

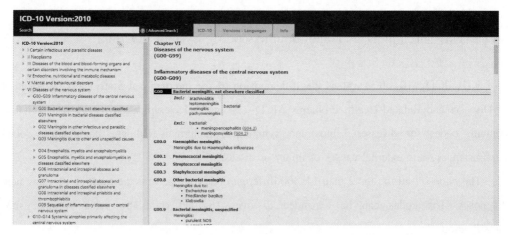

Figure 10‑2　Detailed code and information

Unfortunately, in ICD − 10, besides hierarchy and codes, one can barely find detailed definition for each concept.

3. 2 ICD − 11 (frozen version) WHO is currently revising the ICD towards the ICD − 11. The development is taking place on an internet-based system, called iCAT (Collaborative Authoring Tool) Platform. WHO organized experts of all related fields to contribute to the revision of ICD − 11.

The final draft of the ICD − 11 is expected to be submitted to WHO's World Health Assembly (WHA) for official endorsement by 2019. The peer review was completed in 2018, and the frozen version is available online. It is announced as the final version which will be approved and officially released during WHA 2019.

Over the past several years, WHO has made a major effort to promote traditional medicine across the globe. The inclusion of traditional medicine into the ICD − 11 has the potential to open up doors for its integration into the mainstream medical record keeping and billing systems. The ICD − 11 assists in creating a standardized database for traditional medicine-producing terminologies and classifications for diagnoses and interventions, which are the primary source of health care for many people in parts of Asia, Africa and Latin America as well as Europe and North America.

WHO believes that the use of herbal medicines, acupuncture, and the other traditional medicine practices is significantly increasing during past decades, but due to the absence of related international classifications, this data cannot be collected and compared internationally.

The traditional medicine chapter in ICD − 11 is based largely on the work of the International Classification of Traditional Medicine (ICTM) project experts, who represent a broad spectrum of traditional medicine knowledge from around the world. Many of the experts come from the People's Republic of China, Japan, Republic of Korea, Australia, United States, United Kingdom, Netherland, and some other countries.

Experts who participated in the peer review may also make proposals for revision of ICD − 11, either to address missing content, or to provide updates based on new understanding and information. Through this process, WHO intends to draw upon the broadest possible group of individuals with healthcare expertise to ensure the most accurate up-to-date information possible.

The potential benefits of the formation of International Classifications of Traditional Medicine include the following:

3. 2. 1 Link Traditional Medicine (TM) practices with global norms and standards

development.

3.2.2　Enhance the international public health task on global statistics, surveillance, and public safety.

3.2.3　Support research on TM throughout the world from bench to bed.

3.2.4　Help to give equal access to global public goods for all WHO 193 member states.

3.2.5　Integrate TM into global statistics.

3.2.6　Facilitate the reimbursement for TCM health care.

All in all, there are several new features in this version. Besides, codes and hierarchy, for each concept there will be a short definition. Ontology-based content models have been designed so that experts could define each concept with those models. In this case, in the near future, all the codes, definitions, classifications and hierarchies will be comprehensively understood by computer system. With this intelligent network, experts can easily get data, and make good use of them.

One of the most important new features in ICD - 11 is the TM chapter. It is a stand-alone chapter dealing with TM which at this stage refers to traditional Chinese medicine. In future, other forms of TM will join ICD family. Due to the limited space for a chapter, only limited entities have been included in the TM chapter of ICD - 11. However, the whole framework of TCM diagnosis has been introduced into the chapter. Hopefully, in the near future, the whole value set of TCM diagnosis will be available in the monograph of ICTM project.

With the link below, you can easily access the ICD - 11 Beta browser (Figure 10 - 3). http：//apps.who.int/classifications/icd11/browse/f/en.

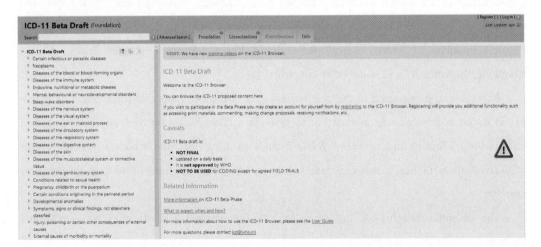

Figure 10 - 3　The UI of ICD - 11 beta browser

3.3 Double coding system in China Currently in China, in TCM hospitals and related departments, we are using a coding system which has been called double-coding system. In this system, doctors are using ICD - 10 to code most of the so-called western diagnosis, ICD - 9 CM3 to code procedures, and the TCD to code TCM diagnosis. TCD codes are also known as GB (Guo Biao, national standards for TCM diagnosis) codes. GB95 is mainly about the classifications and coding of TCM diagnosis, including diseases and patterns. GB97 is mainly about clinical terminologies. When we are making TCM diagnosis, there are two necessary parts: One part is the codes for diseases or disorders, the other part is the codes for patterns. The official revisions of those two standards are at peer review stage. It is believed that the new version of the two GB will be released and put into practice soon.

4. How to Retrieve Diagnosis in ICD Online (Take ICD - 11 as Example)

4.1 Case A 60-year-old female patien, who was diagnosed diabetes mellitus 3 months ago is experiencing thirsty and polyuria. Although drinking a lot, she still has dry mouth and throat. She is also easily agitated and has night sweat. The examination revealed that her tongue is red and scanty fluid with thin yellow coating and her pulse is wiry.

4.2 Procedure

4.2.1 Open a web search. Take Baidu (www.baidu.com) as an example, as shown in Figure 10 - 4.

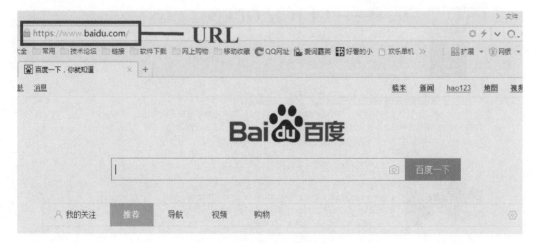

Figure 10 - 4 Baidu search page

4. 2. 2 Input "ICD‑11 WHO" in the search bar, as shown in Figure 10‑5.

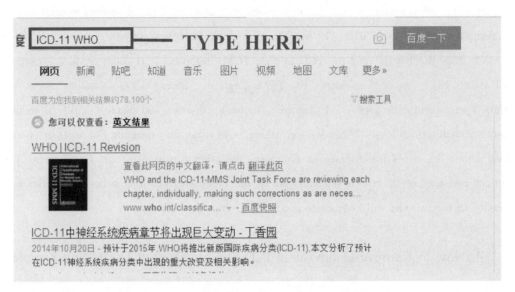

Figure 10‑5 Input "ICD‑11 WHO" in the search bar

4. 2. 3 Click "WHO | ICD‑11 Revision", as shown in Figure 10‑6.

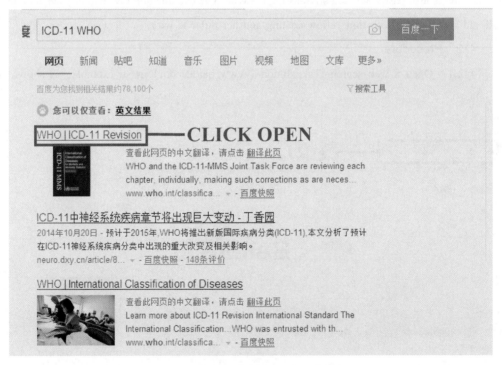

Figure 10‑6 Click "WHO | ICD‑11 Revision"

4.2.4　Search for disorder codes of TCM, as shown in Figure 10 – 7.

4.2.4.1　First click "27 Traditional Medicine conditions — Module I".

4.2.4.2　Second click "Qi, blood and fluid disorders (TM)".

4.2.4.3　Third click "TD71 Wasting thirst disorder (TM)".

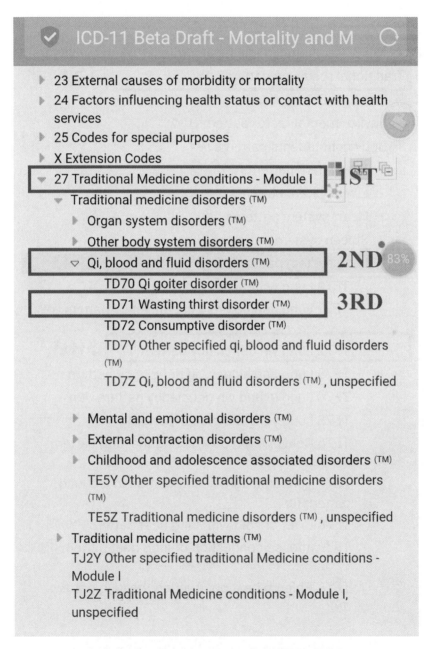

Figure 10 – 7　Result: Its disease code of TCM is TD71

4. 2. 5   Search for pattern code of TCM, as shown in Figure 10 − 8.

4. 2. 5. 1   First click "Traditional Medicine patterns (TM)".

4. 2. 5. 2   Second click "Lung system patterns (TM)".

4. 2. 5. 3   Third click "TF72 Lung yin deficiency pattern (TM)".

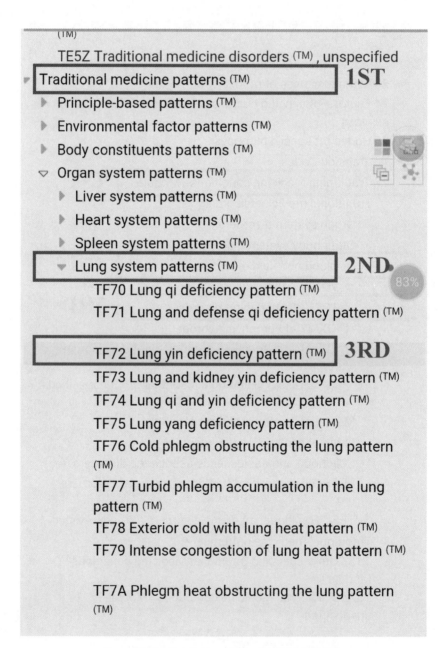

Figure 10 − 8   Result: Its pattern code of TCM is TF72

4.2.6 Search for disease code of Western medicine, as shown in figure 10 - 9.

In this case, we can type "diabetes" in the search bar and we can see much relevant information below.

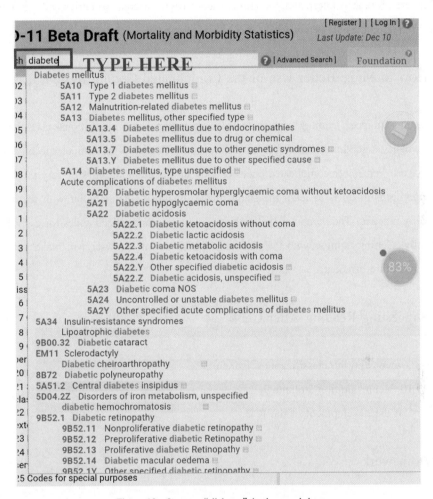

Figure 10 - 9 type "diabetes" in the search bar

5. The Function of International Classification of Disease

If coding standards are different, one cannot group and compare data derived from different countries or area. However, using the same coding standards, data comparison and analysis is made much easier. That is to say, ICD has the potential to assist in unification, standardization, internationalization and convenience.

In current information-based society, ICD accelerates the speed of import and search which could significantly improve health care provider's work efficiency. Moreover, it has a positive meaning in medical record management and clinical scientific research. Also, ICD could promote the health care providers' international communication from different countries and different areas resulting in great contributions for world medical development.

6. How to Make Better Use of the Complicated Coding System

As medical trainee, learning some knowledge on national and international classifications of diagnosis will lay a good foundation for your future work. Thanks to the computer technology, one does not have to remember complicated codes or look up them among piles of very thick books.

All one needs to do is to learn the standardized diagnosis, get familiar with them and use them in daily practice. The computer system helps to assign standardized codes for each diagnosis automatically. Getting familiar with the database of ICD and its browser will make your coding job easier and more efficient.

7. Suggesting Reading After Class

http://www.who.int/classifications/icd/en/.

ICD - 10 Second Edition Volume 2.

History of the development of the ICD.

8. Homework

A 37-years-old male who has gastritis, now has dull epigastric pain, feels oppressed in the chest, dry mouth, no desire to drink, sticky sensation in the mouth, nausea, occasional vomiting. His tongue is red with greasy yellow coating and the pulse is slippery and rapid pulse.

Please search its TCM disease and pattern code, and western disease code.

References

[1] World Health Organization. International Classification of Diseases (ICD) [EB/OL]. [2014 - 02 -

12]https：//www.who.int/classifications/icd/en/.

［ 2 ］ World Health Organization. About WHO［EB/OL］. （2014 − 03 − 14）［2014 − 02 − 09］. https：//www.who.int/about/en/.

［ 3 ］ World Health Organization. The WHO Family of International Classifications［EB/OL］. （2014 − 03 − 14）［2013 − 12 − 22］ https：//www.who.int/classifications/en/.

［ 4 ］ World Health Organization. For the ICD − 11 revision：The ICD 11th Revision is due by 2017［EB/OL］.［2014 − 02 − 17］. http：//www.who.int/classifications/icd/revision/en/.

［ 5 ］ World Health Organization. History of the development of the ICD［EB/OL］.［2020 − 10 − 21］. https：//www.who.int/classifications/icd/en/HistoryOfICD.pdf.

［ 6 ］ World Health Organization. International health statistics using this system are available at the WHO Statistical Information System （WHOSIS）［EB/OL］.［2020 − 11 − 15］. https：//www.who.int/whosis/en/.

［ 7 ］ World Health Organization. International health statistics using this system are available at the Global Health Observatory （GHO） and the WHO Statistical Information System （WHOSIS）［EB/OL］.［2020 − 11 − 17］. https：//www.who.int/data/gho/.

［ 8 ］ Centers for Disease Control and Prevention. ICD − ICD − 10 − CM — International Classification of Diseases［EB/OL］［2015 − 12 −02］. Tenth Revision, Clinical Modification. https：//www.cdc.gov/nchs/icd/icd10cm.htm.

［ 9 ］ U.S. Department of Health & Human Services. HHS Proposes Adoption of ICD − 10 Code Sets and Updated Electronic Transaction Standards［EB/OL］.［2008 − 10 − 22］. https：//en.wikipedia.org/wiki/U.S._Department_of_Health_&_Human_Services.

［10］ World Health Organization. International Classification of Diseases （ICD）［EB/OL］.［2010 − 11 − 23］. https：//www.who.int/classifications/icd/en/.

［11］ ICD − 10 Version. ICD − 10 online browser［EB/OL］.［2015 − 12 − 20］. https：//icd.who.int/browse10/2015/en.

［12］ World Health Organization. ICD − 10 training tool［EB/OL］.［2010 − 12 − 25］. https：//apps.who.int/classifications/apps/icd/icd10training/.

［13］ ICD − 10 Version. ICD 10 Online Support［EB/OL］.［2015 − 12 − 23］. https：//sites.google.com/site/icd10onlinetraining.

附录
一 中医药会议报告书写

在相关专业期刊中,我们可以看到全世界每年都举办各种生物医学及相关领域的学术会议。在这些学术会议上发表的当前医学研究的最新成果,是广大医务工作者获得前沿信息的好方法。它在促进科研成果获得、医务工作者经验交流和培训、促进医学发展方面发挥了重要作用。

一、概述

会议报告的重点是以最简洁的方式,如PPT和海报,向与会者介绍会议内容,吸引各领域的医务人员参加会议,提升会议报告的影响力。本章节介绍的主要内容是参会流程,会议演讲要点,会议PPT和会议海报制作要点等。

二、学习目标

(1)了解会议报告书写格式。

(2)熟悉报告演讲要点。

(3)能够撰写会议报告。

三、参会流程

1. **明确参会目的**　随着科学的发展和信息交流的需求,越来越多的国际专业学术会议出现,形式也越来越广泛。专业学术会议因其有代表性、信息集中化、权威性等特点,引起了医务人员的广泛关注。参与会议的目标如下。

（1）了解当前该领域的主要趋势，进一步把握前沿研究动向，直接获取真实信息。

（2）通过与演讲者和参会人员的积极交流，有助于资源交互，建立合作关系，以及促进科研工作的发展。

（3）通过会议公开并交流研究成果，得到同行的认可和指导，以达到信息共享、促进共同进步和发展的目的。

2. 如何参加会议

（1）收集会议相关信息：随着互联网的日益普及，许多会议信息都发布在互联网上。因此，在互联网检索会议信息方便快捷，与此同时一些专业网站会为有需要的人收集各种有关医学会议的信息。例如：① 卫生部门、中华医学会、各个专业协会和正规的医疗机构发布的通知。② 专业期刊发表在通讯和新闻中的信息。③ 在不同的专业网站获取消息，甚至可以在网上注册。因此定期浏览相关网站，可以及时获得国际和国内医学会议的最新资讯。④ 其他方式。与相关专家进行联系和交流；参加会议可以有机会获得下一次会议的相关信息。

（2）会议材料准备：根据会议信息衡量是否具备参会条件，除了自己的研究内容外，还需要围绕会议中感兴趣的话题发表观点。如果能够顺利注册，我们可以及时与主办方联系，并根据会议要求准备文章。这些材料可以制作成幻灯片或海报来进行展示。

（3）资金准备：注册成功后，你可以选择申报基金来参加相关的专业学术活动，并有机会开展相关临床和科研项目。

3. 材料内容　在学术会议上，所需材料根据会议的目的和形式不同而有所不同。在隆重的会议上发言材料可能是以报告或演讲的形式呈现。两者之间的区别如附表 1 - 1。

附表 1 - 1　会议报告和演讲的联系与区别

对象		报告	演讲
联系		某一与会议主题相关的研究的概述	
区别	内容	结果评价	研究的完成情况，以及经验教训
	重点	研究结果	研究核心内容的承载能力
	表达	简明，客观	科学，生动

四、幻灯片准备

国际会议是国际学术交流的重要形式。15~20分钟的学术报告是会议的主要活动内容。在有限的时间内,演讲者除了口头汇报外,还需借助PPT向参会人员介绍研究的目的、方法,并展示研究结果。

优秀的PPT设计首先需要内容完整,其次是能够帮助演讲者向参会人员展示完整而准确的研究内容。由于学术报告的PPT是对学术论文的概述,因此,与学术论文一样,它是科学研究或临床试验的再现过程。

1. PPT 基本结构

(1)根据 C Slade(1997)学术论文 IMRAD(引言-方法-结果和讨论)的一般结构,PPT演讲的大纲可总结如下:① 摘要:研究目的和背景。② 文献综述:相关研究介绍。③ 研究内容:尽可能使用简短的语句,用词应该贴近读者;注意不同部分的逻辑表达,尽量使用陈述句;确保研究内容不同于摘要或自我主张;尽量避免使用参考文献、表格和缩写;尽量避免使用化学结构式、数字下标和希腊符号;研究内容应该注重研究的创新性和重要性;尽量包含论文的要点和重要的细节(重要的争议或数据)。④ 结果和讨论。⑤ 总结。⑥ 参考文献。

参考文献的书写格式应该符合 GB7714—2015 参考文献著录规则。一般参考文献格式如下。

1)期刊

[序号] 作者.题目[J].期刊名,出版年份,卷号(期号):页码.

e.g. [1] Heider, E.R.& D.C.Oliver. The structure of color space in naming and memory of two languages [J]. Foreign Language Teaching and Research, 1999, (3): 62 - 67.

2)专著

[序号] 作者.题目[M].出版地:出版社,出版年:起始页码.

e.g. [2] Gill R. Mastering English Literature [M]. London: Macmillan, 1985: 42 - 45.

3)论文集

[序号] 作者.题目.[C].主编.论文集名.出版地:出版社,出版年:起始页码.

e.g. [3] Spivak, G. "Can the Subaltern Speak?" [C]. In C. Nelson & L. Grossberg (eds.). Victory in Limbo: Imigism. Urbana: University of Illinois Press, 1988, pp.271 - 313.

4)学位论文

[序号] 作者.题目[D].保存地:保存单位,年份.

e.g. ［4］Almarza, G.G. Student foreign language teacher's knowledge growth［D］. In D. Freeman and J.C. Richards（eds.）. Teacher Learning in Language Teaching. New York：Cambridge University Press, 1996, pp.50－78.

5）报告

［序号］作者.题目,［R］.报告地：主办单位,年份.

e.g.［5］Liming Lu. Quality of reporting and its correlates among randomized controlled trials on acupuncture for cancer pain：Application of the CONSORT 2010 Statement ［R］. Shanghai：World Federation of Chinese Medicine Societies cancer Specialized Committee,2014.

6）专利文献

［序号］专利所有者.专利题目［P］.专利国别：专利号,发布日期.

e.g.［6］Xizhou Jiang. Preparation method of warm external application medicine［P］. China：881056078, 1983－08－12.

7）国际和国内标准

［序号］标准代号,标准名称［S］.出版地：出版社,出版年份.

8）报纸文章

［序号］作者.题目［N］.报纸,出版日期（版次）.

9）电子文献

［序号］作者.题目［文献类型/载体类型］电子文献的出版或可获得地址,发表/更新日期/引用日期（任选）.

（2）不同于传统摘要格式（IMRD 格式），PPT 呈现的摘要格式是一种很好的形式，它更适合科学研究的展示，它可以更加完整、直观地解释实验数据。具体格式如下：① 目的：提出问题、研究目的或假设。② 设计：基本试验设计,样本的选择。③ 大小：研究样本数量。④ 患者,受试者：研究对象的信息。⑤ 干预：处理方法。⑥ 主要观察指标：试验过程。⑦ 结果：该研究的主要发现。⑧ 结论：潜在的应用价值。

2. PPT 制作技巧

（1）保持所有页面整洁：一个严谨的会议报告不需要非常生动地显示界面和眼花缭乱的动画效果。可以充分利用网上一些商务模版,或者 Office 最新版的内容。

（2）合理利用表格：一个好的演讲通常会展示大量的实验或临床数据,通过制作好的表格去展现尤为重要。抑或是在演讲的某一阶段,通过分类表格进行讲解,可以使汇报内容更加清晰、严谨。

（3）正确标注参考文献：会议报告中的任何数据都是公开展示的,对于其中引用的文献需要进行标注,以显示其专业性。并且避免直接侵权行为。

此外,最好要感谢主要参与者。

五、海报制作

国际会议是当前国际学术交流的主要形式之一,会议海报是最重要的交流手段之一。国际会议海报会在会议的指定时间段进行展示(通常是整天),作者需要在特定的时间(通常是几个小时)与感兴趣的参会者进行海报相关的讨论。根据会议规模的不同,海报展示的数量可以从几个到数十万个不等。因此,制作吸引人的海报,反映足够多的信息是实现良好学术交流的重要保证。

总而言之,海报内容应该符合以下要求:表达清晰;研究目的、科学意义和研究假设明确;足够多的结果;恰当的技术;没有额外的技术细节;研究结果能够充分支持结论。

常见的布局如附图 1-1。

题　　目					
作者和隶属单位					
背　　景		结果和讨论			图 ／ 图例
□ 说明 □ □		图	图	图	□ 说明 □ □
		图　　例			
目　　的		图		图例	结　　论
□ 说明 □ □					□ 说明 □ □
材料和方法					参考文献
□ 说明 □ □	图	表格		表格	1. 2.
		图　　例			致　　谢

附图 1-1　海报常见布局

海报举例见附图 1-2。

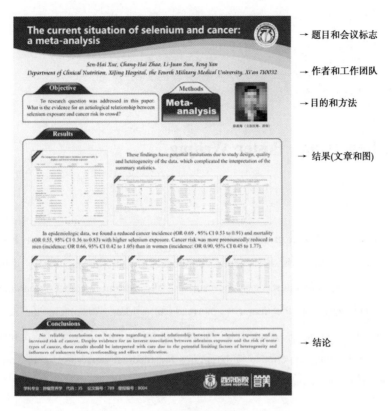

附图1-2 海报举例

六、课后习题

（1）收集一些你感兴趣的国际学术会议的信息。

（2）制作一张海报草图。题目为"人参……的疗效在……人群中的临床研究"。

参考文献

[1] 庄则豪.国际学术会议的壁报制作[J].海峡科学,2009,(11):46-48.

[2] 薛森海.The current situation of selenium and cancer:amata-analysis（8004）[C].第七届中国肿瘤学术大会,2012.

Affiliated One

Meeting Report and Poster Writing

According to the relevant professional journals, each year around the world holds a variety of biomedical and related fields of academic conferences. In this large numbers of the academic conferences, spreading the latest research results of the current medical research and found, which is a good way for the majority of medical workers to obtain the latest medical technology. It has played a great role in promoting scientific research information and achievements, exchanging experience and training for medical personnel in the medical staff, thus promoting the development of medical science.

1. Introduction About This Chapter

The key of the conference report is to present the contents of the conference to the participants in the most concise way, such as PPT and poster, so as to attract medical workers from all sides to participate in the conference and enhance the influence of its report content. In this chapter, some aspects are detailed like participating in the meeting process, meeting speech points, meeting PPT and convention poster making points and others.

2. Objective

To understand the format of paper-writing and reporting of medical meeting.

To be familiar with the main points of the presentation of the report.

Be able to do meeting poster writing.

3. General Registration

3. 1 Why to join in the conference With the development of science and the need of information exchange, more and more international specialized academic conferences have come, and the forms are becoming wider and wider. The professional academic conference is deeply concerned by medical related workers because of its representativeness, information centralization, authority and so on. By participating in the conference, the following objectives can be achieved:

3.1.1 Understand the current main trends in the field, and further grasp the forefront of research directions, direct access to realistic information.

3.1.2 Through the positive communication with speakers and participants, it helps to develop resource interaction, establish cooperative relations, and promote the development of work and scientific research.

3.1.3 Make public the research results, and obtain the approval and guidance of our counterparts through meetings and exchanges so as to achieve the goal of information sharing and mutual promotion and development.

3. 2 How to join in the conference

3.2.1 First of all, we should gather the information about a conference. With the increasing popularity of the Internet, more and more conference information is published on the Internet. So it is easy and fast to retrieve the conference information on the Internet, meanwhile some professional websites collect information on various types of medical conferences for people who need them. e.g., ① Be informed by the health department, the Chinese Medical Association and various professional societies, formal medical institutions. ② According to professional journals published in the newsletter and news. ③ Through the different professional website obtains the news, even can register on the net, therefore searches the related website regularly, then may obtain the newest consultation about the international and domestic medical conference in time. ④ Other ways. Like contacts and private communications with relevant experts; participation in a conference gives you the opportunity to obtain information about the next meeting. So through that way, regularly searching for relevant websites to get the latest information from domestic and international medical conferences.

3.2. 2 Conference material preparation. According to the conference information, to measure whether it is necessary and conditional to attend, in addition to their own research content, but also around the specific topics of interest at the meeting to express their views. If the registration goes well, we can contact the exhibition department in time and prepare the paper according to the meeting requirements. The materials can be made into slides or displayed in the form of posters.

3.2.3　Fund preparation.　After successful registration, you can choose to declare funds to participate in the meeting, in order to choose to participate in related professional academic activities. And having the opportunity to carry out related clinical and research projects.

3.2.4　Content matting.　At an academic conference, the materials required are different depending on the purpose and the form of the meeting. A formal presentation of written material at a solemn meeting could be like a report or presentation, and the difference between the two is as follows (Appendix table 1 - 1):

Appendix table - 1　Similarities and Differences Between Meeting Report and Presentation

Objects		Report	Presentation
Similarities		A general description of the study which meets the topic of meeting	
Differences	Contents	Result evaluation	Completion of the task, achievements and the shortcomings of the work experience
	Emphasis	Project results	The carrying capacity of the core content of the project
	Expression	Concise and objective	Scientific and vivid

4. PowerPoint Preparation

The international conference is an important form of international academic exchange, reading out at the meeting of academic papers is the main activities of the conference, which is in the form of an oral report, usually time for 15 - 20 minutes. To read the paper is to preach and demonstrate parallelly. The speaker in a limited time, in addition to the oral presentation, but also with the help of PPT presentations to the participating counterparts to introduce research purposes and methods, and to demonstrate the results of research.

Excellent design of the PPT script first is to complete the content, then to help the speaker present to the participants with complete and accurate required research information. Due to the academic report of the PPT lecture is a summary of the academic papers, and therefore, as with the academic papers, it is the process of scientific research or clinical trials of reproduction and reflection.

4.1 According to the general structure of C Slade (1997) academic papers IMRD (Introduction-Methodology-Results and Discussion), the outline of PPT lecture notes can be summarized as follows

4.1.1 Abstracts: Research purpose & background.

4.1.2 Literature review: Introduction of related research progress.

4.1.3 Research description: Use short sentences as possible, words should be familiar to potential readers; pay more attention to the logical expression of the different parts, try to use words to express the indicative (level); to ensure the independence of the abstract or self-evident; try to avoid references, charts and abbreviations; try to avoid the use of chemical structure and mathematics of the subscript expressions, and Greek symbols; It should stress the innovation and importance of the research; try to include the main points and important details of the thesis (important arguments or data).

4.1.4 Result presentation and discussion.

4.1.5 Summary and conclusion.

4.1.6 References: The written form shall comply with the Bibliographic references of the GB7714 − 2015. The common references are written in the following format:

4.1.6.1 Periodicals

[serial number] author. document title [J]. journal, year of publication, volume number (issue): page numbers.

e.g. [1] Heider, E.R.& D.C.Oliver. The structure of color space in naming and memory of two languages [J]. Foreign Language Teaching and Research, 1999, (3): 62 − 67.

4.1.6.2 Monographs

[serial number] author. Title [M]. publication: publisher, publication year: start and stop page number.

e.g. [2] Gill R. Mastering English literature [M]. London: Macmillan, 1985: 42 − 45.

4.1.6.3 Collection of papers

[serial number] author. Title of the document. [C]. editor. Title of the paper. Publication: publisher, publication year: start, stop, page number.

e.g. [3] Spivak G. "Can the Subaltern Speak?" [C]. In C. Nelson & L. Grossberg (eds.). Victory in Limbo: Imigism. Urbana: University of Illinois Press, 1988, pp.271 − 313.

4.1.6.4　Dissertation

[serial number] author. Title [D]. save place: save unit, year.

e.g. [4] Almarza, G.G. Student foreign language teacher's knowledge growth [D]. In D. Freeman and J.C. Richards (eds.). Teacher Learning in Language Teaching. New York: Cambridge University Press, 1996, pp.50 – 78.

4.1.6.5　Report

[serial number] author. Title of the literature, [R]. report city: organizer, year.

e.g. [5] Liming Lu. Quality of reporting and its correlates among randomized controlled trials on acupuncture for cancer pain: Application of the CONSORT 2010 Statement [R]. Shanghai: World Federation of Chinese Medicine Societies cancer Specialized Committee, 2014.

4.1.6.6　Patent documents

[serial number] patent owner. Patent title[P]. patent country: patent number, date of issue

e.g. [6] Xizhou Jiang. Preparation method of warm external application medicine[P]. China: 881056078, 1983 – 08 – 12.

4.1.6.7　International and national standards

[serial number] standard code, standard name [S]. publication: publisher, publication year.

4.1.6.8　Newspaper articles

[serial number] author. title [N]. newspaper, publication date (issue).

4.1.6.9　Electronic documents

[serial number] author. Title of electronic document [document type/carrier type] publication or available address of electronic document, publication/update date/reference date (optional).

4.2　Different from the traditional abstract (IMRD format), structured abstract format in the PPT display is also a good way to format which is more suitable for scientific research shows, and it can make the experimental data more perfect and more intuitive The format is outlined below:

4.2.1　Objective: the question, purpose, or assumption of a study.

4.2.2　Design: the basic design of the study, the selection of samples.

4.2.3　Setting: a unit for research.

4.2.4　Patients, participants: information about the object of study.

4.2.5　Interventions: disposal methods.

4.2.6　Main outcome measures: the experimental process.

4.2.7　Results: the main findings of the study.

4.2.8　Conclusions: its potential application.

4. 3　Tips of PowerPoint Making

4. 3.1　Keep all the pages neat: A rigorous conference report does not require a much more vivid display interface and dazzling animation settings, you could find some business type templates on the Internet, or make full use of the latest version of the Office can provide.

4. 3.2　Fair use chart: A good presentation of the general assembly is bound to require a number of experimental and clinical data introduction and presentation. making a good form is particularly important. In the presentation of the stage, use the form of the classification of the introduction, which can make your report clearer and more rigorous style.

4. 3.3　Mark the references correctly: The conference report is a public display in the form of any data on the display in the report, and there should be a description of their quoted references marked, reflecting the professional, but also to avoid direct infringement practices.

Besides, it would be better to thank the main participants.

5. Poster Writing

An international conference is one of the main forms of international academic exchange at present, and the conference poster is one of the most important means of communication. International conference poster at the meeting in the specified time shows (usually all day long), author and poster are required within a specified period of time (usually a few hours) to interested visitors and their poster discussion. According to the different scale of the meeting, exhibition poster numbers could skip from several to hundreds of thousands. Therefore, making the poster attractive, reflecting enough information, is an important guarantee to achieve good academic exchanges.

Overall, the poster content should meet the following requirements: Clear expression; research purpose, clear scientific significance & the research hypothesis; have enough results; the appropriate technology; no extra technical details; results fully support the conclusions; clear and appropriate.

Common layout is as follows (Appendix figure 1 − 1):

Title				
Authors and affiliation				
Background	Results and discussion		Figure	Legend
☐ Captions ☐ ☐	Figure	Figure	Figure	☐ Captions ☐ ☐
	Legend			
Objective				
☐ Captions ☐ ☐	Figure	Legend	Conclusions	
			☐ Captions ☐ ☐	
Material and Methods				
☐ Captions ☐ ☐	Figure	Table	Table	References 1. 2.
	Legend		Acknowledge	

Appendix figure 1 - 1　common poster layout

Poster example（Appendix figure 1 - 2）:

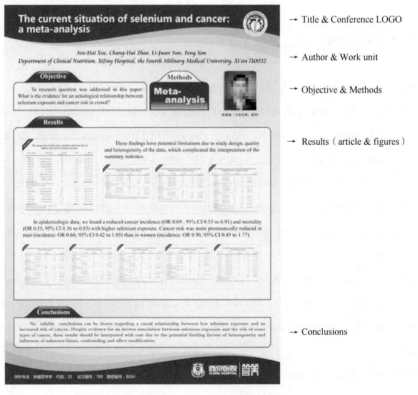

→ Title & Conference LOGO

→ Author & Work unit

→ Objective & Methods

→ Results（article & figures）

→ Conclusions

Appendix figure 1 - 2　Example poster

6. Homework

Homework 1　Gather some information of International academic conference you are interested in.

Homework 2　Make one meeting poster sketch on "Clinical study on the effect of ginseng on ＊ ＊ ＊ in ＊ ＊ ＊ population".

Reference

[1] Zhuang ZH. Poster production for international academic conferences[J]. Straits Science, 2009(11): 46 - 48.

[2] Xue SH. The current situation of selenium and cancer: amata-anlysis (8004)[C]. The 7th Chinese Conference on Oncology, 2012.

中医药研究设计写作与项目撰写

在临床实践过程中,也许你会发现很多临床问题,例如某种治疗方法是否优于另一种治疗方法,如何用循证医学加以证明。此时我们需要设计临床试验。本章节将介绍如何设计研究、不同研究设计种类、适合中医临床研究的研究类型,以及手把手指导如何进行项目撰写。

一、定义

医学研究是一种基础研究,以支持医学领域知识的发展,包括临床研究、临床前研究、基本医学研究。

二、如何开始一项研究

1. 顶层设计

(1)发现临床实践中的问题。例如:患者在术后会有一些并发症,我们能否解决?

研究设计从研究问题开始。你可以通过参加学术会议、阅读文献,或在日常临床经验,发现"限制"或"未来的方向"。

首先,研究问题是你感兴趣的问题。其次,研究问题应具有挑战性和吸引力。第三,研究问题与你的知识密切相关。最后,研究的问题必须是可行的,可以通过实验、观察、调查等解决。一开始可以从简单的研究做起。

(2)科学问题。如果患者服用了某药,我们能否减轻症状?治愈率、有效率、无效率各为多少?

科学的作用是建立一般规律,涵盖有关科学的经验事件或对象的行为,从而使我们能够将事件联系起来,并对未知事件做出可靠的预测。科学问题有助于理论的创新或完善,有助于技术的提高或简化。

(3) 提出假设。比如通过服用某药物,患者的症状可能减轻。

理论建设是一个过程,研究开始通过观察和使用归纳推理,从这些观察得出一个理论(附图2-1)。

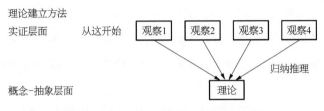

附图2-1 理论建立的方法(归纳法图片示例)

理论测试方法从一个理论开始,用理论指导观察结果: 它从一般到特定。利用演绎推理从理论推导出一组命题(附图2-2)。

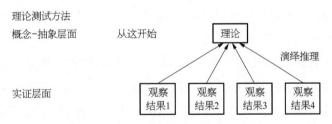

附图2-2 理论建立的方法(演绎法示例)

(4) 建立因果关系模型: 因为患者服用了药物(原因),所以治疗有效(结果)。

2. 研究设计的种类 以下只是突出的几个临床研究类型(包括观察和实验)。若要知道每种研究设计的具体细节,请参考有关讨论研究设计内容的设计研究、临床流行病学和生物统计学相关书或文章。

(1) 系统回顾与 Meta 分析

1) 定义: 系统分析是专注于一个特定的临床问题,通过文献回顾,以验证最优研究方案和总结数据来回答临床问题。这是一个严格的过程。Meta 分析是一个特定类型的系统审查,采用复杂的统计方法(汇集多项小样本研究结果,进行更准确、客观评估的大样本研究)。

2) 优势: 提供当前文献的结构化评论,包括批判性评价的文章;合成许多小的研究,并帮助验证小研究的证据。

3）不足：耗时，研究并不总是很容易地结合起来；临床试验进行分析，必须相似，足以结合；受到原来的研究的偏见影响。

4）举例：Blitz M., Blitz S., Hughes R., et al. (2005). Aerosolized magnesium sulfate for acute asthma: a systematic review[J]. Chest, 128(1): 337-344.

（2）随机对照试验（RTC）

1）定义：真正的实验设计，包括操作干预治疗；研究的参与者被随机分配到实验组或对照组；控制可能是安慰剂或标准治疗；回答问题：干预有什么区别？

2）优势：随机化有助于控制偏倚（组间固有的差异）；对照组的使用提供更好的比较，有助于减轻安慰剂效应；致盲（掩蔽）也可能有帮助；最好建立疗效；提供强有力的因果关系证据。

3）不足：因为伦理问题无法进行某些研究，需要很长的时间，需要健全的方法；昂贵。

4）举例：George J., Raskob G., Vesely S., et al. (2003). Initial management of immune thrombocytopenic purpura in adults: a randomized controlled trial comparing intermittent anti-D with routine care[J]. American Journal of Hematology, 74(3): 161-169.

（3）队列研究

1）定义：从定义的人群（队列）中收集的数据；从暴露、干预或风险因素到结果或疾病进行预期；回答问题：会发生什么？

2）分类：① 前瞻性队列研究：是一个纵向队列研究，随着时间的推移，一组类似的个人（同伙），根据某些因素的研究不同，以确定这些因素如何影响一定的结果发生率。② 回顾性队列研究：是一项纵向队列研究，研究一组个体共享一个共同的暴露因子，以确定其对疾病的发展的影响，并与另一组等效的没有暴露于相同因子的个体进行比较。

3）优势：观察在自然环境中的人；伦理；定时/时间间隔。数据采集提供了可能的结果关联性。比较适合用于中医临床实验设计。

4）不足：没有随机组，可能内在差异（选择偏差）；脱落（参与者退出）可能使结果出现偏差；可能需要长期随访；花费高。

5）举例：Glanz J., France E., Xu S., et al (2008). A population-based, multisite cohort study of the predictors of chronic idiopathic thrombocytopenic purpura in children[J]. Pediatrics, 121(3): e506-512.

（4）病例对照研究

1）定义：回顾时间，从结果或疾病到可能的暴露、干预或危险因素；回答问题：发生了什么？

2）优势：快速和便宜；对具有暴露和结果长时间跨度的罕见疾病有益处；有效的数据一

般来源于记录审查;方便收集及从记录中审查。

3）不足:无随机化;组可能存在内在差异(选择偏倚);难以选择合适的对照组。

4）举例:Berends F., Schep N., Cuesta M., et al. (2004). Hematological long-term results of laparoscopic splenectomy for patients with idiopathic thrombocytopenic purpura:a case control study[J]. Surgical Endoscopy, 18(5): 766 - 770.

（5）病例报告(第八章)

1）定义:描述发生在患者中的观察情况;注意不寻常的关联;注意独特的病例。

2）优势:一个问题的初步观察;新的或罕见的诊断;成本低;可以有进一步的研究。

3）不足:无对照组;无统计有效性;未计划;无研究假设;科学价值有限。

4）举例:Galbusera M., Bresin E., Noris M., et al. (2005). Rituximab prevents recurrence of thrombotic thrombocytopenic purpura:a case report [J]. Blood, 106 (3): 925 - 8.

（6）真实世界研究

1）定义:① 真实世界数据在真实世界环境中,从不同患者群体结局相关的来源中获得的数据,如电子病历、患者调查、临床试验和观察队列研究。② 真实世界证据美国食品及药物管理局定义为"从真实世界数据分析中得出的有关医疗产品使用和潜在利益或风险的临床证据"。③ 真实世界研究对临床常规产生的真实世界数据进行系统性收集并进行分析的研究,是传统循证临床科研以外一种新的采用开放性、非随机、不使用安慰剂的研究类型。从临床试验的实用性出发,从多个数据集(如电子病历、医疗索赔、患者相关信息等)中挖掘信息。

2）优势:① 在各种典型的实践环境中,评估疗效(干预措施所能达到的治疗作用的大小)而非效力(药物自身的一般特征)。② 比较多个替代性干预措施,如老药与新药对比,或除了安慰剂对照组之外有更优的临床策略。③ 数据无法用于随机对照试验的情况。④ 评估新干预的风险效益情况,包括长期临床效益和危害……

3）在中医药领域中的运用:真实世界研究关注具有广泛临床意义的指标,如生活质量等,符合中医"整体观念"。真实世界研究纳入排除标准相对宽泛,例如患者可能同时患有其他疾病,各人饮食习惯、生活方式各有不同,患者之间很难达到完全一致,但均可以作为真实世界研究观察对象。不采用盲法,而根据患者意愿并结合实际医疗条件采取干预措施,符合中医"辨证论治"。

4）不足:概念较新,存在一定争议。相关技术方法有待完善,目前仅作为药品和医疗器械审批决策的补充证据。

5）举例:以人群为基础的甲状腺癌患者死亡概率的预测和评价研究。

（7）其他研究类型：单病例随机对照试验、历史对照研究、不同剂量对照、诊断性病历对照试验……

3. 选择研究类型

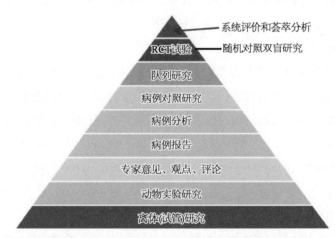

附图2-3　循证证据是临床用药的重要参考依据

（1）证据级别（附图2-3）

1）美国预防服务工作小组（USPSTF）1998：① Ⅰ级：从至少一个合理设计的随机对照试验获得的证据。② Ⅱ-1级：从合理设计的没有随机的对照试验获得的证据。③ Ⅱ-2级：从设计合理的队列或病例对照分析研究获得的证据，从多中心或研究小组进行的试验为佳。④ Ⅱ-3级：从多时间序列设计（有干预手段或无干预手段均可）获得证据。来自无对照组的试验的引人注目的实验结果也被归为此类。⑤ Ⅲ级：权威专家基于临床经验提出的意见。

2）牛津大学EMB中心关于文献类型的新五级标准证据力强、设计严谨、偏差少：① 1a：随机对照试验的系统评价。② 1b：个体的随机对照试验。③ 1c：全或无随机对照试验。④ 2a：队列研究的系统评价。⑤ 2b：个体的队列研究或较差随机对照研究。⑥ 2c："结果"研究；生态学研究。⑦ 3a：病例对照研究的系统评价。⑧ 3b：个体的病例对照研究。⑨ 4：病例系列研究。⑩ 5：未经明确讨论或基于生理学、实验室研究或"第一原则"的专家意见。

3）临床研究的分类（附图2-4）

4）中医临床研究的特点：① 方剂复合成分。② 中医治疗基于辨证论治。③ 中医临床研究设计类型的优化。

中医临床研究根据研究目的，选用不同类型设计。① 中医临床探索性研究过程多选用横断面研究、叙述性研究（如病例报告、病例分析等）设计。② 验证性研究多选用随机对照

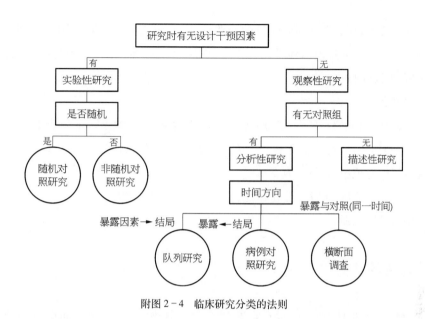

附图2-4 临床研究分类的法则

试验设计。随机对照试验最常用于治疗性或预防性研究,方法比较成熟。随机交叉试验设计,应考虑顺序效应的影响,双盲法是最佳选择。③ 队列研究因为不涉及随机分配患者和盲法,在中医临床研究中可用多种干预措施。病例-对照研究适应面宽,但偏倚较多。④ 横断面研究是中医证候调查常用设计方法。⑤ 叙述性研究是中医临床经验总结、中医探索性研究的常用设计方法。随机方法推荐第三方中央在线网络随机系统,可靠性高,随机化不易被破坏,注重随机隐藏。在不能采用盲法时,盲态测评也可减少测量偏倚,阳性对照必须有高级别证据的支持。⑥ 安慰剂使用可提高循证证据级别。

(2)一步步来:考虑临床、科学问题的阶段。根据特定阶段选择合适的研究设计方法。

1)探索性研究——提出问题:这一阶段的主要任务是提出问题,并初步探索这一问题是否真的是有潜力的科学问题。因此对于这一阶段,我们要以更低的成本、更快的速度得到结论。可使用回顾性的研究设计方案、病例对照研究、病例系列研究。

2)培育性研究阶段——进一步评价治疗效果:在培育性研究阶段,我们通常已经拿到了初步的证据,认为之前提出的概念(科学问题)很可能是成立的。因此我们需要更精确的对效应大小进行估计。此时我们着眼于更高的内部真实性、更少的偏倚,以及相对较高的证据等级。在这一阶段,回顾性队列研究、前瞻性队列研究或是小规模单中心的 RCT 都是我们优先选择的研究方案设计类型。

3)验证性研究——最终验证:这一阶段主要解决上述科学问题的最终验证问题。因此这一阶段的重要目的就是——获取尽可能最高的证据等级。同时,在验证阶段,我们除了关注内部真实性之外,还会关注研究结论的外推能力。因此在这一阶段,多中心的研究也变得更为常见。也可运用大规模队列研究、多中心 RCT、系统综述、临床注册研究等方法。

（3）资源：病例和资金。

4. 研究设计

（1）研究计划：PICO 要素。① P：患者。研究对象,包括纳入标准、排除标准。② I：干预措施（自变量）。独立变量的干预。③ C：比较。对照组。④ O：结果（应变量）,测量结果应客观、科学、有说服力、可重复。

（2）临床研究原则：随机、重复、对照。

（3）临床试验注册。

三、论文的结构[13]

1. 标题 简短且有信息量（少于 25 字）。比如：① Study（analysis/observation/evaluation/assessment）of（on）… by（using…/with…）. ② Effort of A on B. ③ Correlation（relation/relationship）between A and B. ④ Use of … in the treatment of …（illness）in …（piont）.

2. 摘要写作贴士

（1）目的

1）格式：目的,或背景+目的。

2）背景：现在时（一般现在时、完成时、进行时）。

3）目的：一般现在时、完成时、过去式。

比如：The role of omeprazole in triple therapy and the impact of Helicobacter pylori resistance on treatment outcome are not established. This study investigated the role of omeprazole and influence of primary H. pylori resistance one radication and development of secondary resistance.

（2）方法书写贴士

1）纳入标准：… were entered into/enrolled in/selected（randomly）. e.g. A total of 169 patients were included in the study, 83 of whom received …

2）排除标准：… were excluded from participation, with drew from the study due to/because to. e.g. …Patients with significant aortic valvular diseases were excluded.

3）分组：① … were divided into/classified/grouped into. ② … were divided randomly/randomized into. ③ … were divided equally into.

4）研究对象书写贴士：① 年龄：a. Patients（age 26±3 years）. b. Patients under/less than 50 years. c. Patients range in age from … to … with a mean of（50 years）. ② 性别：a. twelve patients（7 male and 5 female）. b. The male-to-female ratio was 1：4. ③ 测定时间：a. Body weight was measured weekly, and liver. b. biopsy was obtained at 4, 8 and 12 weeks.

5）诊断书写贴士：① Be diagnosed as having … ② Be diagnosed as … by …/with … ③ Be suspected as …

6）治疗书写贴士：① Be treated with …（alone or in combination with …）② Be treated on outpatient/inpatient basis. e. g. Patients（n = 539）with a history of duodenal ulcer and a positive H. pylori screening test result were randomized into 4 groups. OAC group received 20 mg omeprazole …

（3）结果书写贴士

1）表达：① The results showed /demonstrated /revealed /documented /indicated / suggested … that … ② A was related/correlated/associated with B. There was a relationship/ correlation between A and B. There was a relation of A with B and C. ③ Increase from … to … with a mean/average（increase）of … ④ increase from … to … with an overall increase of … ⑤ Increase by 3 fold（times）; a 3-fold increase.

2）统计学术语：①（Very/highly）significant difference. ② Insignificant difference. ③ Nonsignificant difference/no difference. ④ There was/is significant difference in … between A and B. ⑤ The difference in … between A and B was/is significant. ⑥ A was/is significant difference from B in … ⑦ No significant difference was found/observed/noted in … between A and B. e. g. There were no significant difference between treatment groups in symptoms and lung function（$P>0.05$）.

（4）总结

1）时态：① 过去时态用于本研究的内容、研究的内容和过程,得出的结论只适合本研究的条件和环境。② 现在时态用于指示描述、前瞻性描述、普遍接受的思想、理论和结论,结论具有普遍意义。如 Our findings indicate that hepatitis C is a progressive disease, but only a few died during the average 20. 4 years after the initiation of injection drug use. Antiviral treatment to eradicate the virus and halt the progression of diseases is indicated in this group of patients.

2）写作贴士：① The results showed/demonstrated/revealed/documented/indicated/ suggested … that … ② A was related/correlated/associated with B. There was a relationship/ correlation between A and B. There was a relation of A with B and C. ③ Increase from … to … with an overall increase of … ④ These results（fail to）support the idea that … ⑤ There is no evidence that … ⑥ Be of great（some/little/no）clinical significance in … to … ⑦ It is remains to be proved that.

3. 引言——解释研究范围和目的　包括一般领域或历史的问题，重要性或需要，以前的研究结果，报告或研究引文可能需要，目前的研究目的和具体领域的问题进行研究。

4. 材料与方法　结果可重复性，方法可操作性，逻辑性。

（1）研究设计：回顾性、前瞻性、临床、动物、实验、跟踪调查、对照、随机、双盲、流行病学等。

（2）研究对象：包括研究对象、分组随机分配的方法、研究组的准入标准、药品或试剂（商标、制造商及其所在地）、测量方法和统计分析方法。在这一部分，我们应该用过去时态。

5. 结果　客观的。包括结果的概述，统计意义，统计支持（图表，表格，照片）。

6. 讨论　与之前的研究比较，展示此次研究的意义。

（1）包括背景，一般研究结果，介绍点，比较的背景，其他研究，建议的意义，结论和未来的研究。

（2）时态：① 确定的结果——现在时；不确定的假设——过去式。② 他人研究成果——过去式或现在完成时。③ 你的研究结果——现在时。④ 众所周知的结论——现在时。⑤ 只适用本研究的结论(过去时)的区别等。

（3）可用的连接词：however，may，might，could，would，possibly，probably，be likely to we believe（think/consider）that，to our knowledge，in our experience（practice）…

7. 致谢　自拟。

8. 参考文献　具体样式参考杂志社规定。比如：

Vega KJ，Pina I，Krevsky B．Heart transplantation is associated with an increased risk for pancreatobiliary disease［J］．Ann Intern Med，1996，124（11）：980－983．

The Cardiac Society of Australia and New Zealand．Clinical excise stress testing：Safety and performance guidelines［J］．Med J，1996（164）：282－284．

9. 插图说明　插图说明需要在其他页面上用双行打印。

10. 插图、表格　插图要按杂志的版面大小比例进行压缩。表格要作为一个独立的信息单位另页打印。

11. 照片与说明　照片要按杂志规定的像素提供，并配以图片说明。

四、研究项目的条目

（1）研究背景。

（2）研究目的。

（3）实验设计：类型、原则、步骤。

1）研究设计类型：小规模、单中心、RTC。

2）实验设计原则：包括病例数、研究方法（随机、对照、盲法等）。

3）研究步骤。

（4）病例选择：包括诊断标准、排除标准、纳入标准。

（5）治疗：包括研究药物名称、说明，药物储存、联合用药。

（6）观察项目：包括项目一般记录和观察点。

（7）观察不良事件：包括不良事件定义、治疗及中止。

（8）疗效和安全性评价标准：包括治疗和继发疗效评价标准和不良事件的程度判断标准。

（9）质量控制与保证的试验：包括实验室质量控制措施、观察指标标准操作规程、培训人员在临床试验前的培训、完善受试者的遵医措施和质量控制和质量保证体系。

（10）知情同意书。

五、阅读材料

（1）Epidemiology, quality and reporting characteristics of systematic reviews of Traditional Chinese Medicine interventions published in Chinese journals.

（2）History of the method ii. Retrospective cohort studies.

（3）《柳叶刀临床研究基本概念》，王吉耀主译。

（4）Framework for FDA's Real-World Evidence Program.

（5）Using real-world data for coverage and payment decisions：The ISPOR real-world data task force report.

六、课后习题

（1）阅读一篇你感兴趣的随机对照试验论文或系统综述。

（2）完成一项你感兴趣的临床研究项目的撰写。

参考文献

［1］百度文库.如何提出研究问题和研究假设［EB/OL］.［2017－04－14］. https://wenku.baidu.com/

view/fa362fd377232f60ddccale7.html.

［2］卡努,安妮·麦考利.科学的局限性：科学方法的哲学批判［J］.人文社会科学学报,2015.20(7)：77－87.

［3］百度文库.什么是研究设计［EB/OL］.［2017－04－08］.https://wenku.baidu.com/view/fe246078a26925c52cc5bfa4.html.

［4］雷切尔·谢尔曼,史蒂文·安德森,杰拉尔德·达尔·潘,等.真实世界证据——它是什么且能告诉我们什么?［J］.新英格兰医学杂志,2016,375(23).2293－2297.

［5］美国食品药品监督管理局.真实世界证据指导原则［EB/OL］.［2019－06－20］.https://www.fda.gov/drugs/webinar-framework-fdas-real-world-evidence-program-mar-15－2019.

［6］吴一龙,陈晓媛,杨志敏.真实世界研究指南［M］.北京：人民卫生出版社,2019.

［7］路易斯·加里森,彼得·诺伊曼,彭尼弗·埃里克森,等.使用真实世界数据进行覆盖和支付决策：ISPOR 真实世界数据工作小组报告［J］.健康价值,2007.10(5)：326－335.

［8］漆舒娴,张宏,刘晓春.真实世界研究及其在中医中的应用［J］.临床医学进展,2018,8(8)：679－682.

［9］舒尔茨·肯尼思,格里姆斯·大卫.柳叶刀临床研究基本概念手册［M］.荷兰：爱思唯尔科学健康科学出版社,2006.

［10］田元祥,翁维良,陆芳.中医临床研究样本量设计的优化［J］.中华中医药杂志,2010,25(5)：710－715.

［11］临床流行病学和循证医学.阶段、资源、证据等级,临床研究方案设计类型你选对了么［EB/OL］.［2018－11－20］.http://mp.weixin.qq.com/s/A4LsrjQZnbD9X1fRHn_Qug.

［12］英国哥伦比亚大学急救医学中心.临床研究：正在开始［EB/OL］.［2007－10－8］.https://www.ubc.ca/research/.

［13］上海译境翻译.医学英语论文写作翻译框架［EB/OL］.［2018－11－10］.http://mp.weixin.qq.com/s/uaI3LPfciapc2cdIO2Ds3A.

Appendix Two

TCM Research Design and Project Writing

You may find many clinical questions like whether a kind of treatment is better than another one during clinical practice. How to prove it by using evidence based medicine? We need to design clinical trials first. This chapter will introduce how to design a clinical research, the different types of research design, research types suitable for TCM clinical research, and teach you how to write projects step by step.

1. Definition

Medical research is a basic research conducted to help and support the development of knowledge in the field of medicine, which includes clinical research, pre-clinical research, and basic medical research.

2. How to Get Start a Research

2.1 Top level design

2.1.1 Questions in clinical practice: For example, The patient may had some kinds of complication after surgery, could we find a way to solve it?

The research design starts with a research question. You may raise research questions by attending an academic meeting, and find "limitations" or "future directions" discussions when reading articles, or during daily clinical experiences.

First of all, the research problem is a question you interested in. Secondly, it's challenging and appealing. Thirdly, it is closely related with your knowledge. At last, the research question must be feasible, which can be solved by experiments, observation, surveys, etc. For beginners, they should start with a simple research problem.

2.1.2　Scientific problem：For example，If the patient took drugs，could the syndrome be relieved? How about the curative rate，the effective rate and adverse events rate?

The function of science is to establish general laws covering the behaviour of empirical events or objects with which the science in question is concerned，and thereby to enable us to connect events，and to make reliable prediction of events as yet unknown. The scientific question makes for the innovation and improvement of theories，as well as the improvement and simplification of technology.

2.1.3　Hypothesis：A research hypothesis is the statement created by researchers when they speculate upon the outcome of a research or experiment.

Every true experimental design must have this statement at the core of its structure，as the ultimate aim of any experiment.

The hypothesis is generated via a number of means，but is usually the result of a process of inductive reasoning where observations lead to the formation of a theory. Scientists then use a large battery of deductive methods to arrive at a hypothesis that is testable，falsifiable and realistic.

For example：The syndrome may be relieved after the patient took the XX（drug）.

Theory building is a process in which research begins with observations and uses inductive reasoning to derive a theory from these observations（Appendix figure 2 – 1）.

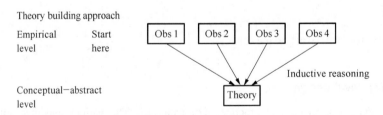

Appendix figure 2 – 1　Method of theory building（example of method）

A theory testing approach begins with a theory and uses theory to guide which observations to make；it moves from the general to the particular. Using deductive reasoning to derive a set of propositions from the theory does this（Appendix figure 2 – 2）.

2.1.4　Establish causal relation model：For example，The patient took the drug（cause），so the therapeutic was effective（effect）.

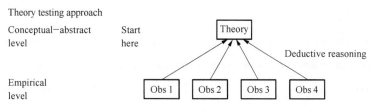

Appendix figure 2 - 2　Method of theory building (example of deductive method)

2.2　Types of research design　The following are just a few highlights of several clinical research types (including observational and experimental). For details on each of them and other types of research design, please consult books on research design/clinical epidemiology/biostatistics or articles discussing research design.

2.2.1　Systematic review and meta-analysis

2.2.1.1　Definition: Systematic review is focusing on a specific clinical topic, conducting a thorough review of the literature, validating best studies and summarizing the data to answer the clinical question. It's a rigorous process.

A meta-analysis is a specific type of systematic review that uses complex statistical methodology (pooling data from individual studies as if one large study).

2.2.1.2　Advantages: Provide structured review of current literature; include articles that are critically evaluated; synthesize many small studies and help validate evidence from small studies.

2.2.1.3　Disadvantages: Very time consuming; studies are not always easily combined; clinical trials to be analyzed must be similar enough to combine; subject to bias from original studies.

2.2.1.4　For example: Blitz M., Blitz S., Hughes R., et al. (2005). Aerosolized magnesium sulfate for acute asthma: a systematic review[J]. Chest, 128(1): 337 - 344.

2.2.2　Randomized controlled trial (RCT)

2.2.2.1　Definition: True experimental design includes manipulating a therapeutic intervention; Participants in the research are randomized to experimental or control groups; Control may be placebo or standard treatment; Answer the question: Does the intervention make a difference?

2.2.2.2　Advantages: Randomization helps control for bias (inherent differences among groups); use of control groups provides better comparison, helps mitigate placebo effect; blinding (masking) when possible also helps; it is best for establishing efficacy; provide strong evidence of causality.

2.2.2.3　Disadvantages: Not possible for some kinds of research that may present ethical dilemmas; Take a long time; Require sound methodology; Expensive.

2.2.2.4　For example: George J., Raskob G., Vesely S., et al. (2003). Initial management of immune thrombocytopenic purpura in adults: a randomized controlled trial comparing intermittent anti-D with routine care[J]. American Journal of Hematology, 74(3): 161 - 169.

2.2.3　Cohort study

2.2.3.1　Definition: Data collected from a defined group of people (cohort) ; look forward in time, from an exposure, intervention, or risk factor to an outcome or disease; answer the question: What will happen?

2.2.3.2　Category: Prospective cohort study: is a longitudinal cohort study that follows over time a group of similar individuals (cohorts) who differ with respect to certain factors under study, to determine how these factors affect rates of a certain outcome.

Retrospective cohort study: is a longitudinal cohort study that studies a cohort of individuals that share a common exposure factor to determine its influence on the development of a disease, and are compared to another group of equivalent individuals that were not exposed to that factor. Retrospective cohort studies have existed for approximately as long as prospective cohort studies.

2.2.3.3　Advantages: Observe people in a natural setting; Ethical; Timing/time intervals of data collection provided possible associations of results. It is suitable for TCM clinical research design.

2.2.3.4　Disadvantages: No randomization; Groups with possible inherent differences (selection bias); Attrition (participant dropout) may bias results; May require long follow-up; Expensive.

2.2.3.5　For example: Glanz J., France E., Xu S., et al (2008). A population-based, multisite cohort study of the predictors of chronic idiopathic thrombocytopenic purpura in children [J]. Pediatrics, 121(3): e506 - 512.

2.2.4　Case control study

2.2.4.1　Definition: Look backward in time, from an outcome or disease to a possible exposure, intervention, or risk factor; answers the question: What happened?

2.2.4.2　Advantages: Quick and cheap; Good for rare disorders with a long time between exposure and outcome; Efficient-data often collected from record reviews; Convenient (patient already have disease).

2.2.4.3 Disadvantages: No randomization; Groups with possible inherent differences (selection bias); Difficult to choose appropriate control group.

2.2.4.4 For example: Berends F., Schep N., Cuesta M., et al. (2004). Hematological long-term results of laparoscopic splenectomy for patients with idiopathic thrombocytopenic purpura: a case control study[J]. Surgical Endoscopy, 18(5): 766 – 70.

2.2.5 Case series/case report (Chapter 8)

2.2.5.1 Definition: Describe observations that have occurred in a patient or a series of patients; Call attention to unusual association; Bring attention to a unique case.

2.2.5.2 Advantages: Preliminary observation of a problem; New or rare diagnosis; Low cost; Can lead to further studies.

2.2.5.3 Disadvantages: No control group; No statistical validity; Not planned; No research hypothesis; Limited scientific merit.

2.2.5.4 For example: Galbusera M., Bresin E., Noris M., et al. (2005). Rituximab prevents recurrence of thrombotic thrombocytopenic purpura: a case report[J]. Blood, 106(3): 925 – 928.

2.2.6 Real world study

2.2.6.1 Definitions

2.2.6.1.1 Real world data(RWD) in medicine is data derived from a number of sources that are associated with outcomes in a heterogeneous patient population in real-world settings, such as Electronic Health Records(EHRs), patient surveys, clinical trials, and observational cohort studies.

2.2.6.1.2 Real world evidence(RWE) is defined by FDA as "clinical evidence regarding the usage and potential benefits or risks of a medical product derived from analysis of RWD".

2.2.6.1.3 Real world study is a systematic collection and analysis of real world data generated by clinical routine. It is a new type of research besides traditional evidence-based clinical research with study design of open, non-randomized and placebo-free. Starting from the practicability of clinical trials, information is mined from multiple data sets (e.g., electronic medical records, medical claims, patient-generated data.).

2.2.6.2 Advantages

2.2.6.2.1 Estimates of effectiveness(the therapeutic effect of interventions) rather than efficacy (general characteristics of drugs) in a variety of typical practice settings.

2.2.6.2.2　Comparison of multiple alternative interventions such as older vs. newer drugs, or clinical strategies to inform optimal therapy choices beyond placebo control group.

2.2.6.2.3　Data in situations where it's not possible to conduct an RCT.

2.2.6.2.4　Estimates of the risk-benefit profile of a new intervention, including long-term clinical benefits and harms ...

2.2.6.3　Application in the field of TCM: Real world research focuses on indicators of wide clinical significance, such as quality of life, which conforms to the "holistic concept" of TCM. The inclusion and exclusion criteria for real world studies are relatively broad. For example, patients may suffer from other diseases at the same time, dietary habits and lifestyles of patients are different. It is difficult to achieve complete identical among patients, however they can all be enrolled for real world studies. Interventions are taken according to patients' willingness and actual medical condition rather than blinding, which is in line with the "syndrome differentiation and treatment" of TCM.

2.2.6.4　Disadvantages: New concept being with controversial. Relevant methodology need to be improved. Now it is a supplementary evidence only used for decision-making on approval of drugs and medical devices.

2.2.6.5　For example: Yang L, Shen W, Sakamoto N. Population-based study evaluating and predicting the probability of death resulting from thyroid cancer and other causes among patients with thyroid cancer[J]. Journal of Clinical Oncology: Official Journal of the American Society of Clinical Oncology, 2013, 31(4): 468.

2.2.7　Other kinds of research types: Single case randomized controlled trial, historical control, dose comparison, diagnostic test case-control ...

2.3　Choose research type

2.3.1　Level of evidence (Appendix figure 2 - 3)

2.3.1.1　The United States Preventive Services Task Force (USPSTF) came out with its guidelines (based on the CTF) in 1988.

Level Ⅰ: Evidence obtained from at least one properly designed randomized controlled trial.

Level Ⅱ-1: Evidence obtained from well-designed controlled trials without randomization.

Level Ⅱ-2: Evidence obtained from well-designed cohort or case-control analytic studies, preferably from more than one center or research group.

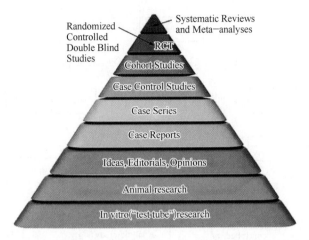

Appendix figure 2 - 3   Evidence-based evidence is an important reference for clinical medication

Level Ⅱ - 3: Evidence obtained from multiple time series designs with or without the intervention. Dramatic results in uncontrolled trials might also be regarded as this type of evidence.

Level Ⅲ: Opinions of respected authorities, based on clinical experience, descriptive studies, or reports of expert committees.

2.3.1.2   Oxford Centre for EBM Levels of Evidence (2009)

1a: Systematic reviews (with homogeneity) of randomized controlled trials.

1b: Individual randomized controlled trials (with narrow confidence interval).

1c: All or none randomized controlled trials.

2a: Systematic reviews (with homogeneity) of cohort studies.

2b: Individual cohort study or low quality randomized controlled trials (e.g. <80% follow-up).

2c: "Outcomes" research; ecological studies.

3a: Systematic review (with homogeneity) of case-control studies.

3b: Individual case-control study.

4: Case series (and poor quality cohort and case-control studies).

5: Expert opinion without explicit critical appraisal, or based on physiology, bench research or "first principles".

2.3.1.3   The classification of clinical researches (Appendix figure 2 - 4)

2.3.1.4   The characteristics of TCM research

2.3.1.4.1   The decoctions are multicomponent, complex intervention.

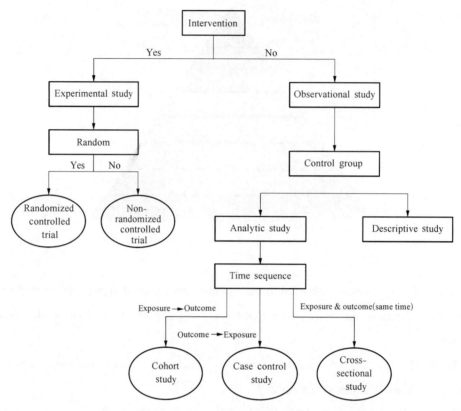

Appendix figure 2 - 4 Classification rules for clinical research

2.3.1.4.2   TCM treatment is based on syndrome differentiation.

2.3.1.4.3   Optimization of design types in TCM clinical research

TCM clinical research covers different design types on the basis of objective of the study. a. For exploratory research of TCM, cross-sectional study and descriptive research (e.g., case report and case analysis) are suitable. b. For hypothesis-testing research, RCT design is commonly adopted. RCT is most commonly used in activity or prevention therapy research, when using randomized cross-over design, the influence of sequence effects should be considered of, and double-blind method is the best choice. c. Cohort study includes various intervention measures, as it doesn't involve randomized allocation and blinding. Case-control study is widely applicable, but it may bring about bias. d. Cross-sectional study is much used in syndrome investigation of TCM clinical research. e. Descriptive research is available for summarization of TCM clinical experience and TCM exploratory research. Third party-central randomization system is recommended, as the randomization is not easy to be damaged. Randomization concealment should also be attached importance. When blinding is impossible, blindness testing could reduce measurement bias, positive control should be supported for high-level evidence. f. Placebo application could improve the level of evidence-based medicine.

2.3.2 Step by step: Take clinical and scientific problems into consideration. Choose proper research and design method according to specific stage.

2.3.2.1 Explorative study-raises a question: The main task of this phase is to raise questions and explore whether the question is really a potential scientific problem. So in this stage, we need to draw conclusions by lower cost and faster speed. Retrospective study design, case control study and case series study are preferred.

2.3.2.2 Cultivation research-further evaluation of therapeutic effects: In this phase, we have a preliminary evidence that the previously concepts (scientific problems) are likely to be valid. Therefore, we need to estimate the effect more precisely. At this point, we should focus on higher internal validity, less bias, and relatively high levels of evidence. Retrospective cohort study, prospective cohort study or small scale single center RCT is preferred.

2.3.2.3 Validation study-final verification: This stage mainly solves the final verification of the scientific problems mentioned above. Therefore, the important purpose of this phase is to obtain the highest level of evidence. At the same time, we will pay attention not only to the internal validity, but also the extrapolation of research results. Therefore, multicenter studies are common at this stage. We can also use large scale cohort study, large scale RCT, systematic review, etc.

2.3.3 Resources: Cases and funds.

2.4 Research design

2.4.1 Research plan: The four PICO elements[12]:

P: Patients. Intended patients/subjects are to study, including the inclusion criteria and exclusion criteria.

I: Intervention (independent variable). The independent variable of interest, intervention and exposure.

C: Comparison. Comparison group or procedure.

O: Outcome (dependent variable). Outcome measurement should be objective scientifical, persuasive and repeatable.

2.4.2 The principal of clinical research: random, repeatable, and control.

2.4.3 Clinical research registry.

3. The Structure of Medical Papers

3. 1　Title　short and concise（less then 25 words）and informative. for example：
a. Study（analysis/observation/evaluation/assessment）of（on）… by（using…/with…）
b. Effort of A on B. c. Correlation（relation/relationship）between A and B. d. Use of … in the treatment of …（illness）in …（point）.

3. 2　Abstract writing tips

3. 2. 1　Objective/purpose/aim.

3. 2. 1. 1　Format：Aim, or background + aim.

3. 2. 1. 2　Tense：Background-present tense（simple present tense, perfect tense, progressive tense）

Aim-simple present tense, perfect tense or past indefinite tense.

3. 2. 1. 3　Example：The role of omeprazole in triple therapy and the impact of Helicobacter pylori resistance on treatment outcome are not established. This study investigated the role of omeprazole and influence of primary H. pylori resistance on eradication and development of secondary resistance.

3. 2. 2　Methods writing tips

3. 2. 2. 1　Inclusive criteria：… were entered into/enrolled in/selected（randomly）. e.g. A total of 169 patients were included in the study, 83 of whom received …

3. 2. 2. 2　Exclusion criteria：… were excluded from participation, with drew from the study due to/because to. e.g. …Patients with significant aortic valvular diseases were excluded.

3. 2. 2. 3　Groups：a. … were divided into/classified/grouped into … b. … were divided randomly/randomized into … c. … were divided equally into …

3. 2. 2. 4　Research objects writing tips：a. Age：a）Patients（age 26±3 years）. b）Patients under/less than 50 years. c）Patients range in age from … to… with a mean of（50 years）. b. Gender：a）twelve patients（7 male and 5 female）. b）The male-to-female ratio was 1 : 4. c. Time of intervention：Body weight was measured weekly, and liver biopsy was obtained at 4, 8 and 12 weeks …

3. 2. 2. 5　Diagnosis writing tips：a. Be diagnosed as having … b. Be diagnosed as … by …/with … c. be suspected as …

3. 2. 2. 6　Treatment writing tips：a. be treated with …（alone or in combination with …）

b. be treated on outpatient/inpatient basis. e.g. Patients($n = 539$) with a history of duodenal ulcer and a positive H. pylori screening test result were randomized into 4 groups. OAC group received 20 mg omeprazole ...

3.2.3　Results writing tips

3.2.3.1　Expressions: a. The results showed/demonstrated/revealed/documented/indicated/suggested ... that ... b. A was related/correlated/associated with B. There was a relationship/correlation between A and B. There was a relation of A with B and C. c. Increase from ... to ... with a mean/average (increase) of ... d. Increase from ... to ... with an overall increase of ... e. Increase by 3 fold (times) ; a 3-fold increase

3.2.3.2　Statistical terms: a. (Very/highly) significant difference. b. Insignificant difference. c. Nonsignificant difference/no difference. d. There was/is significant difference in ... between A and B. e. The difference in ... between A and B was/is significant. f. A was/is significant difference from B in ... g. No significant difference was found/observed/noted in ... between A and B. e.g. There were no significant difference between treatment groups in symptoms and lung function ($P>0.05$).

3.2.4　Conclusion

3.2.4.1　Tense: a. Past tense used in the contents of this research, contents and process of others' researches, and the conclusion only fit this research's condition and environment. b. Present tense used in indicative description, prospective description, universality received thoughts, theories and conclusions, and the conclusion of this research is of universal significance. e.g. Our findings indicate that hepatitis C is a progressive disease, but only a few died during the average 20.4 years after the initiation of injection drug use. Antiviral treatment to eradicate the virus and halt the progression of diseases is indicated in this group of patients.

3.2.4.2　Writing tips: a. The results showed/demonstrated/revealed/documented/indicated/suggested ... that ... b. A was related/correlated/associated with B. There was a relationship/correlation between A and B. There was a relation of A with B and C. c. increase from ... to ... with an overall increase of ... d. These results (fail to) support the idea that ... e. There is no evidence that ... f. Be of great (some/little/no) clinical significance in ... to ... g. It is remains to be proved that ...

3.3　Introduction — to explain the research scope and aim　Including general area or history of problem, importance or need, previous findings, reports or studies citations may be needed, purpose of current study and specific area of problem to be studied.

3. 4 Materials and methods — The reproducibility of the results, manipuility of methods, logicality

3. 4.1 Study: design/protocol, retrospective/review, prospective, clinical, animal, experimental, follow-up, controlled, random/randomized, double-blind crossover, epidemiological, etc.

3. 4.2 Subject: including study objects, methods of any random assignment of subjects to groups, criteria for admission to study groups, drug or reagent (trademark, manufacturer and its location), method of measurement and method of statistic analysis. In this part, we should use the past tense.

3. 5 Results should be described objectively Including the overview of the results, statistical significance, statistical support (charts, tables, photos).

3. 6 Discussion-comparing the previous researches, to show the significance of your research

3.6.1 Including: Background, general findings, introduction of points, comparison in the context of other studies, suggested meaning, conclusion and future studies.

3.6.2 Tense: Certain outcome-present tense; Uncertain of hypothesis-past tense; Others' research results-past tense or present perfect tense; Your research results-present tense; Universal conclusions-present tense; Conclusions only used in this research-past tense.

3.6.3 The conjunction or sentences you can use: However, may, might, could, would, possibly, probably, be likely to, we believe (think/consider) that, to our knowledge, in our experience (practice) …

3. 7 Acknowledgments

3. 8 References-reference styles should be specific to each journal Examples:

3.8.1 Vega KJ, Pina I, Krevsky B. Heart transplantation is associated with an increased risk for pancreatobiliary disease[J]. Ann Intern Med, 1996, 124(11): 980 – 983.

3.8.2 The Cardiac Society of Australia and New Zealand. Clinical excise stress testing: Safety and performance guidelines[J]. Med J Aust, 1996(164): 282 – 284.

3. 9 Legends The legends need to be print in double lines on the other pages.

3. 10 Figures and tables Design your figures for the appropriate reduction.

A table should be a totally self-contained unit of information.

3. 11 Plates and Explanations.

4. Detail List of a Research Protocol

4.1   The research background.

4.2   The purpose of research.

4.3   The experiment design   types, principles and steps.

4.3.1   Research design type (small scale, single center or RCT).

4.3.2   Test design principles: including the number of cases, the research method (random, contrast, blinded, etc).

4.3.3   Test procedure

4.4   Case selection   Including diagnostic criteria, inclusion criteria, exclusion criteria.

4.5   Treatment   Including research drug name and specification, drug preservation and drug combination.

4.6   Observe the project   including project general records and the observation point.

4.7   Observation of adverse events   including the definitions of adverse events, treatment and discontinue of adverse events.

4.8   The curative effect and security evaluation criteria   Including the therapeutic and secondary curative effect evaluation standard and adverse events in degree judgment standard.

4.9   Test of the quality control and assurance   Including the laboratory quality control measures, observation index standard operating procedures, training researchers before clinical trials, improving the subjects compliance measures and quality control and quality assurance system.

4.10   Informed consent.

5. Reading Materials

Epidemiology, quality and reporting characteristics of systematic reviews of Traditional Chinese Medicine interventions published in chinese journals.

History of the method II. Retrospective cohort studies.

The lancet handbook of essential concepts in clinical research by David A. Grimes and Kenneth F. Schulz.

Framework for FDA's real-world evidence program.

Using real-world data for coverage and payment decisions: the ispor real-world data task force report.

6. Homework

Homework 1   Read a randomized controlled trial paper or a systemic review that interests you.

Homework 2   Complete a clinical research project that interests you.

Reference

[1] Wenku Baidu. How to raise research questions and research hypothesis [EB/OL]. [2017 - 04 - 14]. https://wenku.com/view/fa362fd377232f60ddccale7.html.

[2] Kanu, Macaulay A. The Limitations of science: A philosophical critique of scientific method [J]. Journal of Humanities and Social Science, 2015, 20(7): 77 - 87.

[3] Wenku Baidu. What is research design [EB/OL]. [2017 - 04 - 08]. https://wenku. baidu. com/view/fe246078a26925c52cc5bfa4.html.

[4] Sherman RE, Anderson SA, Dal PGJ, etc. Real-world evidence — What is it and what can it tell us? [J]. N Engl J Med, 2016. 375(23). 2293 - 2297.

[5] U. S. Food and Drug Administration. Framework for FDA's real-world evidence program [EB/OL]. [2019 - 06 - 20]. https://www. fda. gov/drugs/webinar-framework-fdas-real-world-evidence-program-mar-15 - 2019.

[6] Wu YL, Chen XY, Yang ZM. A real-world research guide [M]. Beijing: People's Medical Publishing House, 2019.

[7] Garrison LP Jr, Neumann PJ, Erickson P, et al. Using real-world data for coverage and payment decisions: the ISPOR real-world data task force report[J]. Value Health, 2007, 10(5): 326 - 335.

[8] Qi SX, Zhang H, Liu XC. Real world study and its application in the field of traditional Chinese medicine [J]. Advances in Clinical Medicine, 2018, 8(8): 679 - 682.

[9] Schulz K, Grimes D. The lancet handbook of essential concepts in clinical research [M]. Netherlands: Elsevier Science Health Science Div, 2006.

[10] Tian YX, Weng WL, Fang LU. Optimization of design types in TCM clinical research [J]. China Journal of Traditional Chinese Medicine and Pharmacy, 2010, 25(4): 556.

[11] Clinical Epidemiology and Evidence-Based Medicine. Have you chosen the right stage, resources,

level of evidence, and type of clinical research plan? [EB/OL]. [2018 - 11 - 20]. http://mp. weixin.qq.com/s/A4LsrjQZnbD9X1fRHn_Qug.

[12] Medical Center Department of Emergency Medicine of UBC. Clinical research: getting started [EB/OL]. [2007 - 10 - 8]. https://www.ubc.ca/research/.

[13] Transvoice. A framework for translating medical English paper writing [EB/OL]. [2018 - 11 - 10]. http://mp.weixin.qq.com/s/uaI3LPfciapc2cdIO2Ds3A.

附录 三 词汇表

一稿多投	duplicate publication	Chapter 2
癫、狂、痫	psychosis, mania, and epilepsy	Chapter 3
E		
耳穴压豆	seed	Chapter 5
F		
分	Fen	Chapter 1
风轮	wind orbiculi	Chapter 6
敷贴治疗	sticking treatment	Chapter 5
造假	fabrication	Chapter 2
G		
膏方	Gao Fang	Chapter 5
甘草	Licorice	Chapter 1
感冒病	common cold disease	Chapter 3
感受外邪	be suffered from exogenous pathogenic agent	Chapter 3
感受时气之邪，袭于表分，湿热夹滞，互阻肠胃	caught the wind evil while late summer prevailing damp and hot caused hysteresis, damage Wei-Qi, stagnant intestines and stomach.	Chapter 4
共情能力	empathy ability	Chapter 8
桂枝	Cinnamon Twig	Chapter 1
H		
寒哮	cold-wheezing	Chapter 6
寒热往来	alternately felt hot and cold	Chapter 4
黑睛	cornea	Chapter 6
滑石	Talc	Chapter 1
化痰平喘	resolve phlegm, and relieve wheezing	Chapter 6
化湿和胃	dissipating dampness and harmonizing stomach	Chapter 4
怀牛膝	Achyranthes bidentate	Chapter 1
喉中喘鸣气粗，痰色黄	Hot-wheezing: coarse and gurgling wheeze in the throat with sticky yellow phlegm	Chapter 6
喉中如有水鸡声，痰色白	cold-wheezing: frog-croak-like gurgling in the throat with white clear phlegm	Chapter 6
I		
诚信	integrity	Chapter 2

脾虚泄泻	diarrhea（spleen deficiency syndrome）	Chapter 5
平行病历	parallel case	Chapter 8
Q		
欺骗	fraud	Chapter 2
气不摄血	Qi can not control blood	Chapter 5
气关	Qi Guan	Chapter 5
气轮	Qi orbiculi	Chapter 6
气阴两虚	Qi and Yin deficiency	Chapter 5
气短	shortness of breath	
清心丸	Qingxinpill	Chapter 4
情志受伤	emotional injuries	Chapter 3
祛寒消积	warming and purgation	Chapter 4
R		
热盛	excessive heat	Chapter 5
热伤络脉	heat damage the collaterals	Chapter 5
肉轮	flesh orbiculi	Chapter 6
乳积	dyspepsia of milk	Chapter 5
S		
少腹痛	lower abdomen pain	Chapter 4
芍药	Chinese herbaceous peony	Chapter 1
上焦	upper Jiao	Chapter 6
湿热	dampness heat	Chapter 3
湿浊中阻	dampness obstructing the middle	Chapter 4
失眠	insomnia	Chapter 3
四诊合参	TCM four diagnostic methods	Chapter 6
四肢抽搐	twitching in the extremities	Chapter 3
舌白润无苔	tongue is white and wet without coating	Chapter 4
舌质暗红,苔白腻	tongue quality is dark red and coating is white and greasy	Chapter 4
三焦	Sanjiao theory（triple burner）	Chapter 3
神疲体倦	mental and physical lassitude	Chapter 3
生姜	Ginger	Chapter 1
生赭石	Raw sienna	Chapter 1

宣泄情绪	express and control emotion	Chapter 5
血轮	blood orbiculi	Chapter 6
Y		
眼睑	eyelid	Chapter 6
阴	Yin	Chapter 2
阴寒积聚	cold stagnation	Chapter 4
饮食不节	unhealthy diet	Chapter 3
营血炽热	heat penetrating the blood	Chapter 4
语无伦次	incoherent speech	Chapter 3
Z		
躁妄打骂,喧扰不宁,动而多怒	manic agitation with excessive movement and anger	Chapter 3
谵语	ravings	Chapter 3
脏腑	viscera	Chapter 3
真迹	medical record	Chapter 1
真武汤	Zhenwu decoction	Chapter 4
证	Zheng(patterns)	Chapter 1
症	symptom	Chapter 3
治法	therapeutic methods	Chapter 6
中焦	middle Jiao	Chapter 6
中医耳诊	TCM ear diagnosis	Chapter 6
中医病(疾病)和中医证(证候)	TCM Bing(diseases) and Zheng(patterns)	Chapter 9
中医病证分类与代码(简称95国标 GB95)	classification and codes of Diseases and Zheng of Traditional Chinese Medicine(GB95)	Chapter 9
中医临床诊疗术语(简称97国标 GB97)	Clinic Terminology of Traditional Chinese Medicine Diagnosis and Treatment(GB97)	Chapter 9
中医面诊	TCM face diagnosis	Chapter 6
重、浊、腻	heaviness, turbidity, greasy	Chapter 3
铢	Zhu	Chapter 1
主诉	chief complaint	Chapter 3
自我剽窃	self-plagiarism	Chapter 2
自身信誉	self-credibility	Chapter 2
左金丸	Zuojin pill	Chapter 4

Appendix Three

Wordlist

A

achyranthes bidentate	怀牛膝	Chapter 1
adjusting diet	调饮食	Chapter 4
alternately felt hot and cold	寒热往来	Chapter 4
analysis of the disease in etiology and pathology	辨证分析（中医病因及病机）	Chapter 3
aversion to cold and fever	恶寒发热	Chapter 3
aversion to the wind	恶风	Chapter 4
avoiding getting cold	避风寒	Chapter 4

B

be suffered from exogenous pathogenic agent	感受外邪	Chapter 3
Bing（diseases）	病	Chapter 1
blood orbiculi	血轮	Chapter 6

C

canthus	两眦	Chapter 6
caught the wind evil while late summer prevailing damp and hot caused hysteresis, damage Wei-Qi, stagnant intestines and stomach	感受时气之邪,袭于表分,湿热夹滞,互阻肠胃	Chapter 4
chief complaint	主诉	Chapter 3
Chinese herbaceous peony	芍药	Chapter 1
Cinnamon Twig	桂枝	Chapter 1
Classification and codes of diseases and Zheng of Traditional Chinese Medicine（GB95）	中医病证分类与代码（简称 95 国标 GB95）	Chapter 9
Clinic terminology of traditional Chinese medicine diagnosis and treatment（GB97）	中医临床诊疗术语（简称 97 国标 GB97）	Chapter 9
cold stagnation	阴寒积聚	Chapter 4
Cold-wheezing	寒哮	Chapter 6

Cold-wheezing: frog-croak-like gurgling in the throat with white clear phlegm	喉中如有水鸡声,痰色白	Chapter 6
common cold disease	感冒病	Chapter 3
constipation	便结	Chapter 3
cornea	黑睛	Chapter 6
D		
Da Qinglong decoction	大青龙汤	Chapter 4
damp-heat of lower-Jiao	下焦湿热	Chapter 5
dampness heat	湿热	Chapter 3
dampness obstructing the middle	湿浊中阻	Chapter 4
deep and string tight pulse	脉沉而弦紧	Chapter 4
delirium with muscle twitching and cramp	筋惕肉瞤	Chapter 4
diarrhea	痢下	Chapter 4
diarrhea (spleen deficiency syndrome)	脾虚泄泻	Chapter 5
differentiation of disease and syndrome	鉴别诊断(辨病与辨证)	Chapter 3
disease identification	辨病	Chapter 3
dissipating dampness and harmonizing stomach	化湿和胃	Chapter 4
duplicate publication	一稿多投	Chapter 2
dyspepsia of food	食积	Chapter 5
dyspepsia of milk	乳积	Chapter 5
E		
emotional injuries	情志受伤	Chapter 3
empathy ability	共情能力	Chapter 8
excessive heat	热盛	Chapter 5
express and control emotion	宣泄情绪	Chapter 5
external contraction	外感	Chapter 3
eye white	白睛	Chapter 6
eyelid	眼睑	Chapter 6
F		
fabrication	造假	Chapter 2
fainted	猝然昏倒	Chapter 3
falsification	造假	Chapter 2
Fen	分	Chapter 1
Fengguan	小儿指纹风关	Chapter 5

manic agitation with excessive movement and anger	躁妄打骂, 喧扰不宁, 动而多怒	Chapter 3
medical record	真迹	Chapter 1
mental and physical lassitude	神疲体倦	Chapter 3
middle Jiao	中焦	Chapter 6
Mingguan	命关	Chapter 5
more joyful with silence	静不多言	Chapter 6
P		
palpitation	惊悸	Chapter 4
parallel case	平行病历	Chapter 8
pathological indicators	病理特征	Chapter 8
phlegm dampness	痰湿	Chapter 3
physical obesity	形体肥胖	Chapter 3
plagiarism	剽窃	Chapter 2
psychosis, mania, and epilepsy	癫、狂、痫	Chapter 3
pupil	瞳仁	Chapter 6
Q		
Qi and Yin deficiency	气阴两虚	Chapter 5
Qi can not control blood	气不摄血	Chapter 5
Qi orbiculi	气轮	Chapter 6
Qiguan	气关	Chapter 5
Qingxin Pill	清心丸	Chapter 4
quick pulse	脉数	Chapter 4
R		
ravings	谵语	Chapter 3
Raw sienna	生赭石	Chapter 1
reddish urinary	尿赤	Chapter 3
relieving exterior syndrome, dredging stagnant	解表导滞	Chapter 4
resolve phlegm, and relieve wheezing	化痰平喘	Chapter 6
road-opening formula	开路方	Chapter 5
S		
Salami-slicing	萨拉米饼切片式	Chapter 2
Sanjiao theory (triple burner)	三焦	Chapter 3
seed	耳穴压豆	Chapter 5

self-credibility	自身信誉	Chapter 2
self-plagiarism	自我剽窃	Chapter 2
shallow tight pulse	脉浮紧	Chapter 4
shortness of breath	气短	Chapter 3
silent dementia	沉默痴呆	Chapter 3
six-meridians	六经	Chapter 3
small and soft pulse	脉濡细	Chapter 4
soothing liver Qi	疏泄少阳	Chapter 4
sound like pigs and sheep in the mouth	口中如作猪羊叫声	Chapter 3
sputum cover the Qingqiao	痰闷清窍	Chapter 5
stagnation of the water circulation	水液循环停滞	Chapter 6
sticking treatment	敷贴治疗	Chapter 5
stomach Yin deficiency	胃阴不足	Chapter 5
stool was white and red	赤白相杂	Chapter 4
sweat slightly	微汗	Chapter 4
symptom	症	Chapter 3
syndrome identification	辨证	Chapter 3
T		
Talc	滑石	Chapter 1
TCM Bing(diseases) and Zheng(patterns)	中医病(疾病)和中医证(证候)	Chapter 9
TCM ear diagnosis	中医耳诊	Chapter 6
TCM face diagnosis	中医面诊	Chapter 6
TCM four diagnostic methods	四诊合参	Chapter 6
tenesmus	里急后重	Chapter 4
text-recycling	文字再利用	Chapter 2
the evil from Shao Yang depressed into Jue Yin, inversely attack Yang Ming	病从少阳,郁入厥阴,复从厥阴,逆攻阳明	Chapter 4
the GB(Guo Biao, National Standard) on Bing (diseases) and Zheng(patterns)	病和证相关的国标(GB)	Chapter 9
therapeutic methods	治法	Chapter 6
thick coating	苔腻	Chapter 4
thirst without desire for drink	渴不欲饮	Chapter 3
to warm the lung, dispel cold	温肺散寒	Chapter 6
tongue is white and wet without coating	舌白润无苔	Chapter 4

tongue quality was dark red and coating was white and greasy	舌质暗红,苔白腻	Chapter 4
twitching in the extremities	四肢抽搐	Chapter 3
U		
undescending of gastric Qi	胃气不降	Chapter 4
unhealthy diet	饮食不节	Chapter 3
upper Jiao	上焦	Chapter 6
V		
vertex	巅顶	Chapter 4
viscera	脏腑	Chapter 3
vomiting in the mouth	口吐涎沫	Chapter 3
W		
warming and purgation	祛寒消积	Chapter 4
water orbiculi	水轮	Chapter 6
weak pulse	脉弱	Chapter 4
Wei-Qi-Yin-blood	卫气营血	Chapter 3
Wheezing necessarily occurs combined with panting, but panting can occur alone.	喘必兼哮,哮未必兼喘	Chapter 6
wind orbiculi	风轮	Chapter 6
wiry and long pulse on the other	脉右部弦长,按之有力	Chapter 4
X		
Xiaoyao decoction	逍遥散	Chapter 4
Y		
Yin	阴	Chapter 2
Z		
Zhenwu decoction	真武汤	Chapter 4
Zheng(patterns)	证	Chapter 1
Zhu	铢	Chapter 1
Zuojin pill	左金丸	Chapter 4